Prescription guidelines in cardiology

ROBERT HAÏAT

rmer Head of the Cardiology Department
Saint-Germain-en-Laye Hospital
sociate Professor at the Hospitals of Paris
College of Medicine

GÉRARD LEROY

Head of the Cardiology Department
Saint-Germain-en-Laye Hospital
Former Senior Registrar-Assistant
in the Hospitals of Paris

Prescription guidelines in cardiology

2nd edition

Preface by Professor Pierre GODEAU

ÉDITIONS FRISON-ROCHE

By the same authors, from the same publisher:

- Cardiovascular therapeutics: Cross-sectional analysis of the major clinical trials. Preface by Prof. Cl. Guérot, 1999.
- Major clinical trials in cardiovascular therapeutics. Preface by Prof. P. Théroux, 2001.
- Hypertension. Lessons from the major clinical trials, 2004.
- Stable angina and post-myocardial infarction. Lessons from the major clinical trials, 2004.

© Éditions Frison-Roche,18, rue Dauphine, 75006 Paris, 2006, 2009
E-mail: infos@editions-frison-roche.com

Scientific data also available on : www.cardio-log.com

(ISBN 2-87671-498-1 1st edition)

ISBN 978-2-87671-521-9

Preface

There is something fascinating about progress in medicine, particularly in the field of therapeutics. The excessive mediatization of medical knowledge often has perverse consequences by focusing the general public's attention on spectacular aspects, while ignoring the essential aspects of everyday medical practice.

Doctors themselves are increasingly disconcerted and medical decision-making is becoming more and more difficult each day, torn between the often illusory rigor of supposedly scientific evidence, the principle of precaution that tries to rationalize the irrational, and economic constraints. The time may come when, like Buridan's ass, the doctor will be unable to choose between two apparently equivalent options. Replacement of individual decision-making by a collegiate decision often constitutes a progress, but may also conceal paralysis of personal reflection in favor of sharing of responsibilities and risks to minimize the role of the general practitioner, who usually knows his patient, in the Hippocratic meaning of the term, better than other doctors.

Finally, the progressive popularization of Internet access recalls Aesop's judgment: "The tongue is at once the best and the worst of things". Increasingly informed patients are often poorly informed and are unable to separate the good grain from the chaff, a task that is already difficult for the doctor. It is therefore essential for all general practitioners to have a sound knowledge in order to avoid medical errors as far as possible and to be used as a guide to decision-making and this is the purpose of this book "Prescription guidelines in cardiology", which constitutes a model that could be applied to other disciplines. It constitutes a body of verified, evaluated, updated information that will allow all doctors, cardiologists as well as general practitioners, internal physicians and other specialists, to rapidly update their knowledge, as so many of the topics discussed, hypertension, hypercholesterolemia, diabetes, venous disease, stroke, extend well beyond the confines of cardiology and concern all medical specialities. Furthermore, objective information in more specifically cardiological fields will also allow non-specialists to keep up to date with progress in this field, enabling them to actively participate in the decision-making process or to reassure an anxious patient on the basis of objective data rather than simple compassion.

The rapid growth of knowledge often invalidates the results of multicenter studies, which can become obsolete even before their publication. Consensus conferences provide a snapshot of the state of knowledge at a given moment in time rather than an objective guideline.

Another difficulty concerns the complexity of medicine, as the interactions between the various organs are often ignored: the hepatic, muscle, or hematologic toxicity of certain drugs or the consequences of renal insufficiency on a particular drug prescription, etc. Limiting therapeutic trials to typical cases with the preliminary exclusion of unusual cases is certainly an essential criterion to conduct a good quality controlled trial, but it must be remembered that about 25% of patients do not meet these criteria and it is precisely these patients who raise the most difficult problems in clinical practice.

Aware of these difficulties, the experienced practitioner, not straight out of medical school, will find in this book the irreplaceable data that he or she would never have the time to find in a database.

We can only be impressed by the immense task that the authors have set themselves and the clarity of the presentation of this book. The color paragraph headings provide a rapid overview in response to a specific question.

A more detailed reading indicates the studies on which the proposed answer is based. The meticulous or perfectionist reader can then refer to the original publications that are all referenced.

It is exceptional for a medical text to be so well presented and this clearly constitutes an improvement of the medical service provided to doctors. Acquisition of this book is highly recommended for continuing medical education that each practitioner must ensure independently or as a complement to official directives which always remain mysterious and which should have been updated years ago.

Professor Pierre GODEAU
Professor Emeritus of Internal Medicine
Member of the French National Academy of Medicine

Table of contents

Foreword

By paving the way to evidence-based medicine, the major clinical trials published in the international literature have imposed their law and have profoundly modified the therapeutic approach to cardiovascular disease.

As these trials have become the basis for modern medicine, they can no longer be ignored, as this would lead to a risk of not providing patients with the best possible care in line with the most recent scientific data, as required by medical ethics.

However, this is a difficult task for the practitioner. Absorbed by the worries and responsibilities inherent to everyday practice, it is not easy to find a guide to treatment decisions within the increasing volume of often contradictory data.

The ideal solution would be to have a text that highlights the main conclusions of the major trials, a text that presents the essential findings.

We have tried to write such a text based on our experience of more than 20 years in this field. By reviewing essential concepts, defining practical applications, and specifying dosages, we have written a clear and concise vade-mecum that we have enriched, whenever possible, by the most recent guidelines from international scientific societies.

Once again, we hope that we have written a useful book by providing practitioners and students with the main keys to modern cardiovascular therapy.

Robert HAÏAT
Gérard LEROY

Main abbreviations used in this book

ABPM: Ambulatory blood pressure measurement
ACC: American College of Cardiology
ACE: Angiotensin-converting enzyme
ACS: Acute coronary syndrome
ADA: American Diabetes Association
AF: Atrial fibrillation
ARBs: Angiotensin II receptor blockers
BHS: British Heart Society
BMI: Body Mass Index
BNP: Brain natriuretic peptide
BP: Blood pressure
BPM: Beats per minute
DBP: Diastolic blood pressure
EASD: European Association for the Study of Diabetes
ECG: Electrocardiogram
ESC: European Society of Cardiology
Hb: Hemoglobin
HbA1c: glycosylated hemoglobin
HDL: High-density lipoproteins
HDL-C: HDL-cholesterol
HT: Hypertension
INR: International normalized ratio
IV: Intravenous
LDL: Low-density lipoproteins
LDL-C: LDL-cholesterol
LMWH: Low molecular weight heparin
LV: Left ventricular
LVEF: Left ventricular ejection fraction
LVH: Left ventricular hypertrophy
mEq: milliequivalent
mmHg: millimeters of mercury
MMSE: Mini Mental State Evaluation
NICE: National Institute for health and Clinical Excellence
NS: Non significant
NT pro-BNP: N-terminal pro-BNP
NYHA: New York Heart Association
RR: Relative risk
SBP: Systolic blood pressure
SC: Subcutaneous
TEE: Trans esophageal echocardiography
TIA: Transient ischemic attack
U: Unit
UFH: Unfractionated heparin

CHAPTER 1

Hypertension

Factual data

■ Hypertension (HT) is a cardiocerebrovascular risk factor.

  ■ It increases the risk of stroke (particularly ischemic cerebral infarction rather than hemorrhagic infarction) more than the risk of myocardial infarction.

  ■ This concept, not reported in the older meta-analyses by **Mac Mahon** and **Collins**, probably because the criteria of several of the older trials included in these meta-analyses were not sufficiently precise, was revealed by the analysis by **Kjeldsen** and by the **LIFE** study.

■ The increased risk of cardiovascular morbidity and mortality is directly and continuously correlated with blood pressure (BP) beyond a value of 115/75 mmHg.

  ■ This was demonstrated by the **PSC** study based on 61 prospective observational studies including 1 million adults initially free of cardiovascular disease; with a follow-up of 12.7 million subject-years, it confirmed the continuous correlation between cardiovascular risk and blood pressure beyond a diastolic blood pressure of 75 mmHg; a 20 mmHg difference in SBP has the same consequences as a 10 mmHg difference in DBP.

  ■ This continuous correlation between BP and cardiovascular risk does not allow the definition of a precise cut-off value for hypertension.

■ After the age of 50 and especially in elderly patients, systolic blood pressure (SBP) is a better indicator of cardiovascular risk than diastolic blood pressure (DBP).

■ DBP still has a certain prognostic value before the age of 50, as it tends to decrease physiologically after the age of 50-55 years.

■ Treatment of HT improves the cardiovascular prognosis.

■ It has been known since the **Framingham** study that the treatment of HT improves the prognosis of all forms of HT, i.e. malignant hypertension (DBP > 140 mmHg associated with a neurological and/or cardiac and/or renal lesions and/or ocular fundus lesions), severe HT (SBP $\geq$ 180 mmHg or DBP $\geq$ 110 mmHg) or even mild-to-moderate HT (SBP between 140 and 149 mmHg or DBP between 90 and 109 mmHg).

■ In primary prevention, lowering of peripheral SBP/DBP decreases the risk of stroke to a much greater extent than the risk of coronary events.

■ According to the meta-analysis by **Collins**, any antihypertensive therapy able to reduce DBP by 5 to 6 mmHg could decrease the 5-year risk of stroke by 50% and the 5-year risk of coronary events by about 20% (or even 30% beyond 5 years).

■ Antihypertensive therapy improves the prognosis proportionally to the reduction of blood pressure figures.

■ This was demonstrated by the **HDFP**, **HOT** and **BBB** studies.

■ This was confirmed by the **BPLTTC** meta-analysis. In the first cycle of this meta-analysis based on 15 large trials comprising 74,696 hypertensive patients, intense *vs* more moderate antihypertensive therapy significantly reduced the relative risk of stroke by 20%, that of coronary disease by 19% and that of a major cardiovascular event by 15%, without modifying the risk of cardiovascular or all-cause mortality. In the second cycle of this meta-analysis based on 14 large trials comprising 87,669 hypertensive patients, stricter blood pressure control more markedly decreased the number of strokes and all cardiovascular events.

Definitions and diagnosis

Systolic-diastolic hypertension
■ It is defined by an office SBP ≥ 140 mmHg and/or DBP ≥ 90 mmHg.

■ These figures must be confirmed by two measurements at the same visit and on 3 successive visits over a period of 3 months, or within several days or weeks when BP is ≥ 180/110 mmHg.

Isolated systolic hypertension
■ It is defined by SBP ≥ 140 mmHg and DBP ≤ 90 mmHg.

■ It is frequent in the elderly (see p. 32) and, like systolic-diastolic hypertension, is associated with a cardiovascular risk but also an increased risk of dementia.

Pulse pressure
■ It is defined by the difference between SBP and DBP.

■ Any increase of pulse pressure ≥ 60 mmHg (generally corresponding to a combination of high SBP and normal or low DBP) is an independent predictive index of cardiovascular mortality, especially coronary mortality, and stroke.

Central blood pressure
■ This is the pressure exerted on the aorta and thus directly at the organ level: heart, brain, kidneys.

■ Central systolic BP or aortic pulse pressure are measured at the site of "central" arteries like the aorta (central aortic BP) and the common carotid arteries (central carotid BP). Central BP can now be estimated noninvasively from the pressure wave recorded in a peripheral artery.

■ It is sometimes different from the BP measured in the arm; thus, for an identical reduction of brachial BP, some antihypertensives decrease central BP, the while others do not modify central BP.

■ The increase in central BP appears to be a major factor of large and small cerebral artery remodeling (increasing the risk of stroke). The increased left ventricular load is associated with an increased left ventricular mass with a parallel reduction in myocardial tissue perfusion. An increase in central pulse pressure is associated with renal dysfunction (**Laurent** and **Cockroft**). Subsequently, central BP is significantly correlated with the risk of cardiovascular events.

So-called white coat HT (or isolated clinic HT)

■ It is defined as high BP at every office visit in contrast with normal BP on ABPM or self-measurement.

■ It is associated with a lower cardiovascular risk than permanent HT and can be managed simply by lifestyle and dietary measures and regular follow-up.

Masked HT (or isolated ambulatory HT)

■ It is defined by a normal BP in the doctor's office in contrast with high BP on ABPM or self-measurement.

■ It is accompanied by an increased prevalence of target organ damage and metabolic risk factors; the associated cardiovascular risk is similar to that related to permanent HT.

Exercise HT

■ It is defined by an excessive rise in BP during an exercise test or physical (cold pressor test) or mental stress.

■ Its prognostic value has not been clearly demonstrated and it has not been demonstrated to be correlated with the development of permanent HT or target organ damage. Patients should therefore not be systematically screened for exercise HT.

■ Self-measurement of BP and/or ABPM (ambulatory blood pressure monitoring) are now recommended to validate the permanent nature of mild-to-moderate HT (140-179/90-109 mmHg) before initiating treatment, in the absence of high risk.

■ These techniques also allow identification of:

– white coat HT with a good prognosis identical to that of normotensive subjects, but which nevertheless requires regular surveillance;

– masked HT, i.e. normal BP in the doctor's office, but high BP on self-measurement and/or ABPM, defined more recently, which is associated with the same cardiovascular risk as permanent HT.

■ The prognostic value of these techniques is superior to that of BP measurements performed in the doctor's office.

◆ *SBP and DBP cut-off values defining HT are 135/85 mmHg on self-measurement and 130/80 mmHg on 24-hour ABPM.*

■ Once the diagnosis of HT has been confirmed, the patient's global cardiovascular risk must be evaluated.

■ This risk corresponds to the 10-year probability of developing a cardiovascular event.

■ It can be evaluated from the American **Framingham** equation (*JAMA* 2001; *285*: 2486-2497) which evaluates the risk of a cardio-vascular event, or the European **SCORE** system (*Eur Heart J* 2003; *24*: 1601-1610) which evaluates the risk of cardiovascular death.

■ A 10-year risk ≥ 20% according to the **Framingham** equation or ≥ 5% according to the **SCORE** system, indicates a high risk.

Non-pharmacological treatment

■ Non-pharmacological treatment of HT, i.e. weight reduction, increased physical exercise, dietary measures (sodium restriction, increased consumption of fruit, vegetables and potassium), significantly lowers blood pressure, but compliance tends to wane in the long term.

■ Any weight reduction ≥ 4 kg decreases blood pressure.

■ This was demonstrated by the **TAIM, TOHP I, TONE** and **TOHP II** studies.

■ A reduction of sodium intake lowers BP by about 3.5/1.5 mmHg.

■ This was demonstrated by the **TOHP II** and **DASH-Sodium** studies and the meta-analyses by **Midgley** based on 28 trials comprising 1,131 hypertensive patients and **Graudal** based on 58 trials comprising 2,161 hypertensive patients.

■ In practice, it is recommended to limit salt (NaCl) intake to 6 g daily.

■ A diet rich in fruit and vegetables increases potassium intake and improves blood pressure.

- This was demonstrated by the **DASH** study conducted in 459 patients with mild HT with a follow-up of 3 weeks.

- Similarly, the meta-analysis by **Whelton**, based on 33 randomized trials comprising 2,609 hypertensive patients showed that an oral potassium supplement of 60 to 75 mmol daily significantly lowered blood pressure.

■ Lifestyle and dietary measures designed to obtain a multifactorial reduction of risk factors improve BP of hypertensive patients even when they are already treated by monotherapy.

- This was demonstrated by the **DEW-IT** study conducted in 44 obese hypertensive patients treated by monotherapy. With a follow-up of 9 weeks, lifestyle and dietary measures, comprising moderate physical exercise 3 times a week, and a low-calorie and low-salt DASH diet, vs control group achieved a mean weight loss of 4.9 kg and a reduction of SBP (by 9.5 mmHg; $p < 0.001$) and DBP (by 5.3 mmHg; $p < 0.002$) measured by ABPM.

- This was also demonstrated by the **PREMIER** study conducted in 810 patients with a mean age of 50 ± 8.9 years and higher than optimal blood pressure or untreated mild HT (SBP: 120-159 mmHg and DBP: 80-95 mmHg). With a follow-up of 6 months, weight loss of at least 6.8 kg when body mass index was ≥ 25 kg/m^2, sodium intake limited to 100 mEq daily and moderate physical exercise for at least 180 minutes/week associated with a DASH diet achieved an optimal blood pressure (< 120/80 mmHg) in 35% of cases (vs 30% for lifestyle modification only [$p = 0.024$] and vs 19% in the control group which only received advice [$p < 0.001$]).

■ Compliance with non-pharmacological treatment tends to wane with time and becomes poor in the long term.

- This was observed after one year in the **TOMHS** study and after 3 years in the **TOHP II** study.

Pharmacological treatment

■ Five classes of major antihypertensive drugs (diuretics, beta-blockers, calcium channel blockers, ACE inhibitors, ARBs) can be proposed as first-line treatment of uncomplicated essential HT.

■ It has now been demonstrated that these 5 therapeutic categories reduce cardiovascular morbidity and mortality.

■ This is not the case for alpha-blockers and centrally-acting antihypertensives, which are not recommended as first-line therapy, but which can help to achieve the blood pressure goal in the case of adverse effects or from the stage of triple-agent therapy.

Diuretics and beta-blockers

■ For more than 30 years, clinical trials have demonstrated the efficacy of diuretics and beta-blockers.

■ In primary prevention, diuretics and beta-blockers were, for a long time, the only therapeutic categories proven to induce a comparable reduction of morbidity and mortality.

■ This was demonstrated, in particular, by the **MRC** and **HAPPHY** studies and was confirmed by the meta-analysis by **Psaty**.

Diuretics

■ This remains true for thiazide diuretics (chlorthalidone or hydrochlorothiazide) administered at 12.5 to 25 mg daily, which are effective in the prevention of cardiovascular morbidity and mortality.

■ This was the conclusion reached by the meta-analysis by **Psaty** based on 42 trials comprising 592,478 patients, which evaluated 7 therapeutic strategies including placebo.

■ In this meta-analysis, on a head-to-head comparison of monotherapy, no therapeutic category (beta-blockers, ACE inhibitors, calcium channel blockers, ARBs) was found to be significantly more effective than low-dose thiazide diuretics.

■ Indapamide can be included in this therapeutic category, as it is a sulfonamide related to thiazides. Indapamide SR 1.5 mg has a demonstrated antihypertensive efficacy and complies with some international guidelines which recommend the use of low-dose diuretics in the first-line treatment of HT.

◆ *According to the JNC-VII guidelines, thiazide diuretics must be an integral part of the treatment of most cases of uncomplicated HT and HT cannot be considered to be refractory if antihypertensive therapy does not include a diuretic. However, according to BHS-NICE guidelines, diuretics should not be a first line treatment in hypertensives younger than 55 years (see p. 39).*

■ Thiazide diuretics can be usefully coprescribed with a potassium-sparing diuretic.

■ This combination avoids thiazide-induced potassium depletion and could reduce the incidence of sudden death and limit glucose intolerance induced by hypokalemia.

Beta-blockers

■ The efficacy of beta-blockers in primary prevention has recently been questioned.

■ In the meta-analysis by **Lindholm** based on 13 trials comprising 105,951 patients, beta-blockers (half of which being atenolol), compared to other antihypertensives, induced a significant 16% increase (p = 0.009) of the risk of stroke and were not found to be superior in terms of prevention of myocardial infarction or death. These results can be explained by a less marked reduction of central SBP and an increased risk of harmful metabolic effects such as *de novo* diabetes, especially when beta-blockers are associated with diuretics.

■ These findings might not apply to new generation beta-blockers (carvedilol, nebivolol) which possess vasodilator properties but clear proofs are still awaited.

◆ *According to a study by **Messerli**, about 20-25% (i.e. about 250,000 cases) of the one million cases of new-onset diabetes arising yearly in USA could possibly be* *related to the use of the so-called traditional antihypertensive drugs, thiazide diuretics and/or beta-blockers.*

Calcium channel blockers

■ After a persistent controversy arising from the contradiction between the favorable results of most clinical trials and the more reserved results of some meta-analyses, calcium channel blockers have now regained their place in the treatment of HT.

■ These problems essentially concerned first generation dihydropyridines, which were considered to have a proischemic effect due to coronary steal and they also increased heart rate, sympathetic activity and myocardial oxygen consumption.

◆ *According to **JNC-VI** guidelines, verapamil, diltiazem, and third generation dihydropyridines can be used as first-line treatment for HT in the same way as other classes of antihypertensive drugs.*

■ In the **FEVER** study, conducted in China on 9,711 patients with hypertension poorly controlled (SBP: 140-180 mmHg or DBP: 90-100 mmHg) by hydrochlorothiazide 12.5 mg and presenting 1 or other 2 cardiovascular risk factors in addition to HT, addition of felodipine 5 mg daily *vs* placebo, with a follow-up of 40 months, only slightly lowered BP (-3.5/-1.5 mmHg), but significantly decreased the risk of fatal or nonfatal stroke (primary endpoint) by 27% ($p = 0.001$) and the incidence of cardiovascular events by 27% ($p < 0.001$).

■ In the **VALUE** study conducted in 15,245 high-risk hypertensive patients with a mean follow-up of 4.2 years, treatment with amlodipine 5 mg daily was found to be as effective as treatment with valsartan 80 mg daily in the prevention of cardiovascular events (primary outcome) but was significantly more effective on myocardial infarction reduction, one of secondary outcomes (-19%; $p = 0.02$).

Angiotensin-converting enzyme inhibitors (ACE inhibitors)

■ ACE inhibitors improve more the cardiovascular prognosis than the other anti-hypertensive agents.

■ In the **CAPPP** study conducted in 10,985 hypertensive patients who received, under open-label conditions, either captopril 50-100 mg daily associated with a diuretic if necessary, or a beta-blocker or a diuretic (associated if necessary) in order to achieve a DBP < 90 mmHg, captopril demonstrated the same efficacy as the other treatments on BP and on the main composite endpoint of the study (fatal or nonfatal myocardial infarction, fatal or nonfatal stroke and other cardiovascular mortality) with a mean follow-up of 6.1 years, but was associated with an increased risk of nonfatal stroke (Relative risk: 1.25 [1.01-1.55]; p = 0.044).

■ In the **HOPE** study conducted in primary and secondary prevention in 9,297 patients with a mean age of 66 years at high risk of a cardiovascular event (46.8% of subjects included were hypertensive), but not presenting either left ventricular dysfunction or heart failure, the addition of ramipril 10 mg daily *vs* placebo to standard therapy significantly decreased by 22% (p < 0.001) the relative risk of the main composite endpoint (myocardial infarction, stroke or cardiovascular mortality) and each component of this primary endpoint, with a follow-up of 5 years.

■ In the **ANBP 2** study conducted in 6,083 hypertensive patients (mean age: 71.9 years), treatment with enalapril *vs* treatment with hydrochlorothiazide, with a mean follow-up of 4.1 years, significantly decreased the risk of cardiocerebrovascular events or death by 11% (p = 0.05) and the incidence of nonfatal myocardial infarction by 32% (p = 0.04), with no modification of the total number of strokes, which was comparable in the 2 treatment groups.

■ In the **EUROPA** study (see p. 36) conducted in 12,218 patients with coronary disease, 57% of whom were hypertensives, perindopril high dose once daily reduced significantly by 20% (p = 0.0003) the incidence of the primary endpoint (cardiovascular death, nonfatal myocardial infarction and resuscitated cardiac arrest) and major cardiovascular events (fatal and non fatal myocardial infarction [– 24%], and hospitalisation for heart failure [– 39%]).

◆ *ACE inhibitors slow the progression of renal failure (see p. 62).*

■ In the meta-analysis by **Jafar** based on 11 trials comprising 1,860 nondiabetic hypertensive patients with a mean age of 47.5 years and a mean follow-up of 2.2 years, treatment including an ACE inhibitor compared to treatment without an ACE inhibitor reduced proteinuria by an additional 0.46 g/day. This treatment also decreased the relative risk of end-stage renal disease by 31%. A significantly greater benefit of ACE inhibitor therapy was observed in patients with the highest baseline proteinuria.

■ These results were confirmed by the **AASK** study conducted in 1,094 Afro-American patients aged 18 to 70 years with HT complicated by renal disease.

■ In the **ASCOT-BPLA** study (see p. 22) the amlopidine-perindopril based regimen was associated with a significant 15% (p = 0.018) reduction of development of renal impairment.

■ ACE inhibitors decrease the risk of diabetes by about 20%.

■ In the **CAPPP** study conducted in 10,985 hypertensive patients, treatment with captopril 50-100 mg daily compared to treatment with beta-blocker (atenolol or metoprolol 50-100 mg daily) or diuretic (hydrochlorothiazide 25 mg daily or bendroflumethiazide 2.5 mg daily), combined if necessary, significantly reduced the risk of *de novo* diabetes by 14% (p = 0.039).

■ In the **HOPE** study conducted in patients at high risk of cardiovascular disease, ramipril 10 mg/day *vs* placebo decreased by 32% (p < 0.001) the percentage of patients developing diabetes.

■ In the **ALLHAT** study conducted in high risk hypertensive patients, lisinopril 10 to 40 mg/day *vs* amlodipine 2.5 - 10 mg/day decreased by 13% (p < 0.05) the risk of new cases of diabetes.

■ In the **ANBP-2** study conducted in elderly hypertensive patients, enalapril based regimen *vs* conventional therapy decreased by 31% (p < 0.0005) the onset of new cases of diabetes.

■ In the **INVEST** study conducted in 22,576 hypertensive patients with coronary heart disease, trandolapril 2 mg daily and verapamil SR 240 mg daily *vs* atenolol 50 mg daily and hydrochlorothiazide 25 mg daily significantly decreased the incidence of *de novo* diabetes (6.16% *vs* 7.29%) with a mean follow-up of 2.7 years.

■ In the **ASCOT-BPLA** study, conducted in 19,257 hypertensive, amlodipine 5-10 mg daily and perindopril 4-8 mg daily *vs* atenolol 50-100 mg daily and bendroflumethiazide 1.5-2.5 mg daily decreased the incidence of *de novo* diabetes by 30% (p < 0.0001) with a mean follow-up of 5.4 years. According to **Gupta**, given evidence from previous trials, it seems likely that the differential effect of the two antihypertensive regimens used in ASCOT-BPLA on new onset diabetes is a composite of the adverse effects on risk produced by atenolol and thiazide, plus the protective effects of perindopril, with amlodipine probably playing a neutral role.

■ Although it does not invalidate these concepts, it should be noted that, in the **DREAM** study conducted in 5,269 patients without cardiovascular disease (43,3% were hypertensives, however) but with impaired fasting glucose levels or impaired glucose tolerance (43.3% of patients had a history of HT; base line BP: 136 ± 18.6/83.4 ± 10.8 mmHg) and specifically designed to confirm this finding, the use of ramipril (up to 15 mg/day) *vs* placebo for 3 years failed partially to achieve this objective as it did not significantly reduce the incidence of the primary outcome (diabetes or death) but did significantly increase regression to normoglycemia.

◆ *According to the Task Force of the European Society of Cardiology, ACE inhibitors are also the first-line treatment for HT in patients with heart failure, decreased LVEF, diabetes or a high coronary risk.*

Angiotensin II receptor blockers (ARBs)

■ ARBs seem to improve the cardiovascular prognosis.

■ In the **LIFE** study conducted in 9,193 hypertensive patients with ECG signs of LVH, compared to atenolol 50-100 mg daily, losartan 50-100 mg daily, possibly associated with hydrochlorothiazide 12.5-25 mg daily or other antihypertensives in both arms, with a mean follow-up of 4.8 years, significantly reduced the incidence of the primary endpoint comprising cardiovascular death, myocardial infarction or stroke, by 13% (p = 0.021). But only the incidence of fatal and non fatal stroke was decreased by 25 % (p = 0.001) while the incidence of cardio-vascular mortality and myocardial infarction was not reduced. In a *post-hoc* analysis it was also found that losartan decreased *de novo* atrial fibrillation by 33% (p < 0.001), reducing the incidence of stroke by 45% (p = 0.039) in this group (*JACC* 2005; *45*: 705-711). This result was obtained with a similar reduction of BP in the 2 treatment groups.

■ In the **VALUE** study conducted in primary and secondary prevention on 15,245 hypertensive patients (mean age: 67.2 years) with high cardiovascular risk, treatment with valsartan 80 mg daily was found to be as effective as treatment with amlodipine 5 mg daily for the prevention of fatal and nonfatal cardiovascular events (except myocardial infarction), with a mean follow-up of 4.2 years.

■ In the **Jikei Heart** study, an open trial conducted in Japan on 3,081 patients with hypertension, coronary heart disease, heart failure or a combination of these diseases, addition of valsartan 40-160 mg daily (mean dosage: 76 mg daily) to standard therapy *vs* absence of ARBs, with a mean follow-up of 3.1 years, decreased the main composite endpoint comprising cardiovascular morbidity and mortality by 39% (p = 0.0002), essentially due to a significant (p = 0.028) 40% reduction of the incidence of stroke and TIA, a 65% reduction (p < 0.0001) of the incidence of angina and a 47% reduction (p = 0.029) of the incidence of heart failure with no difference for mortality.

■ In the **ONTARGET** study (see p. 25) conducted in patients who had vascular disease or high risk diabetes, telmisartan was not inferior to ramipril in the prevention of major cardiovascular events.

■ In the **MOSES** study (see p. 187) conducted in hypertensive patients with a history of stroke or TIA and treated by eprosartan, a decrease of cardiocerebrovascular risk was also described.

■ ARBs slow the progression of renal failure.

■ This was demonstrated by **IRMA II**, **IDNT** and **RENAAL** studies conducted in diabetic patients (see p. 62, 66-67).

■ ARBs result in some decrease of the risk of diabetes.

■ In the meta-analysis by **Elliott** and **Meyer** based on 22 clinical trials comprising 143,153 patients, mostly hypertensive (17 trials), the incidence of *de novo* diabetes was lowest with ARBs and ACE inhibitors, immediately followed by calcium channel blockers, beta-blockers and diuretics.

■ In the **LIFE** study (see p. 22), treatment with losartan *vs* treatment with atenolol decreased the incidence of *de novo* diabetes by 25% (p = 0.001) with a mean follow-up of 4.8 years.

■ In the **VALUE** study (see p. 23) valsartan 80 mg daily *vs* amlodipine 5 mg daily decreased the incidence of *de novo* diabetes by 23% (p < 0.0001) with a mean follow-up of 4.2 years.

■ In the **ONTARGET** study (see p. 25) new onset of diabetes was slightly higher on telmisartan 80 mg/day *vs* ramipril 10 mg/day (7.5% *vs* 6.7%) but the difference was not statistically significant (RR 1.12 [0.97-1.29]).

■ In the **PRoFESS** study (see p. 187) addition of telmisartan 80 mg once a day *vs* placebo to optimal treatment did not modify the incidence of metabolism and nutrition disorders (2% *vs* 2%).

■ In the **TRANSCEND** study (see p. 25) there were fewer patients in the telmisartan 80 mg/day group exhibiting signs of new diabetes than in the placebo group, although not significantly so (11.0% *vs* 12.8%; p = 0.08).

ACE inhibitors *vs* ARBs

■ The efficacy of ACE inhibitors and ARBs in the prevention of cardiovascular risk has been compared in some studies.

■ In the **BPLTTC** meta-analysis presented by **Turnbull**, no significant difference was observed between ACE inhibitors and ARBs in terms of reduction of the risk of stroke or heart failure. In contrast, ACE inhibitors were found to be significantly (p = 0.001) superior to ARBs in terms of prevention of the risk of myocardial infarction or cardiovascular mortality.

■ The meta-analysis by **Strauss** and **Hall** reached the same conclusions.

■ The recent meta-analysis by **Reboldi** based on 6 trials (including **ONTARGET**) comprising a total of 49,924 patients did not reveal any significant difference between ACE inhibitors and

ARBs in terms of the risk of myocardial infarction (OR 1.01; p = 0.75), cardiovascular mortality (OR 1.03 ; p = 0.23) and all-cause mortality (OR 1.03; p = 0.20). ARBs provided slightly better stroke protection than ACE inhibitors (OR 0.92; p = 0.037). It should be noted that this meta-analysis included also patients taking ARB on top of ACE inhibitor.

■ In the **ONTARGET** study conducted in 17.078 patients who had vascular disease or high risk diabetes without heart failure, telmisartan 80 mg/day was not inferior to ramipril 10 mg/day in the prevention of death from cardiovascular causes, myocardial infarction, stroke or hospitalization for heart failure (16.5% *vs* 16.7%; RR 1.01[0.94 to 1.09]).

■ ARBs can be useful when ACE inhibitors are poorly tolerated as they induce less cough and angioneurotic edema, but are associated with a higher risk of hypotension.

■ This was demonstrated by the **ONTARGET** primary and secondary prevention study conducted in 25,620 patients already receiving optimal therapy; addition of telmisartan 80 mg daily was not inferior to addition of ramipril 10 mg daily in terms of prevention of cardiovascular events (cardiovascular mortality, myocardial infarction, stroke, hospitalization for heart failure), observed in 16.66% *vs* 16.46% of cases (non-inferiority: p = 0.0038) with a mean follow-up of 56 months. Treatment with telmisartan was associated with a significantly lower rate of cough (1.1% *vs* 4.2%) and angioedema (0.1% *vs* 0.3%) but an excess of symptomatic hypotension (2.6% *vs* 1.7%).

◆ Although the **TRANSCEND** study confirmed the good safety of ARBs compared to placebo, it did not demonstrate the efficacy of ARBs in patients intolerant to ACE inhibitors.

■ In the **TRANSCEND** study, conducted in 5,926 patients intolerant to ACE inhibitors with cardiovascular disease or diabetes with target organ damage, with a follow-up of 56 months, the addition of telmisartan 80 mg daily *vs* placebo to baseline therapy reduced BP by 4.0/2.2 mmHg but did not modify the incidence of the primary composite endpoint (cardiovascular mortality, myocardial infarction, stroke or hospitalization for heart failure) observed in 15.7% *vs* 17.0% of cases (p = 0.216).

Telmisartan significantly decreased, by 13% (non adjusted p = 0.048; adjusted p = 0,068), one of this study's secondary end-points (cardiovascular mortality, myocardial infarction or stroke) which was the primary endpoint of the **HOPE** study (see p. 20).

■ When prescribing ACE inhibitors or ARBs, it is recommended to monitor renal function.

■ Serum creatinine and serum potassium must be assayed one to two weeks after starting treatment. Any elevation of serum creatinine by more than 20-30% requires discontinuation of the medication and referral for a specialist opinion.

Alpha-blockers and centrally-acting antihypertensives

■ Alpha-blockers and centrally-acting antihypertensives are not recommended as first-line therapy, as their efficacy for prevention of cardiovascular morbidity and mortality has not been formally demonstrated.

Antihypertensive combinations

■ If the blood pressure goal is not achieved after at least 4 weeks, second-line dual therapy must be instituted.

■ Dual therapy can be started earlier when BP is > 180/110 mmHg regardless of the number of risk factors or when BP is 140-179/90-109 mmHg in a patient with a high cardiovascular risk.

■ Combinations of new therapeutic categories may be more effective than the conventional diuretic-beta-blocker combination.

◆ *In the **ASCOT-BPLA** arm of the **ASCOT** study, the calcium channel blocker-ACE inhibitor combination was superior to the beta-blocker-diuretic combination in the prevention of total and cardiovascular mortality.*

■ In this study conducted in 19,257 hypertensive patients aged 40 to 79 years with at least 3 cardiovascular risk factors and a mean follow-up of 5.4 years, the combination of amlodipine 5-10 mg daily + perindopril 4-8 mg daily *vs* the combination of atenolol 50-100 mg daily + bendroflumethiazide 1.25-2.5 mg daily reduced the relative risk of mortality by 14% (p = 0.005), the relative risk of the composite endpoint comprising coronary mortality, nonfatal infarction, *de novo* angina and heart failure by 14% (p = 0.0048), and cardiovascular mortality by 24% (p = 0.0017), stroke by 23% (p = 0.0007) and *de novo* diabetes by 32% (p < 0.0001). The superiority of this combination appeared to be independent of BP reduction alone. This study made a major contribution to the debate concerning the place of beta-blockers in the current treatment of HT, emphasized the value of antihypertensive combinations and resulted in a modification of BHS-NICE guidelines (see p. 39).

◆ *In the **ACCOMPLISH** study, the benazepril-amlodipine combination was shown to be superior to the benazepril-hydrochlorothiazide combination for cardiovascular risk prevention.*

■ In this study conducted in 11,506 patients (mean age: 68.3 years) with isolated systolic HT (SBP > 160 mmHg) already treated in 97% of cases (by dual therapy in 74% of cases) but controlled (SBP < 140/90 mmHg/) in only 37.5% of cases, with a follow-up of 39 months, the combination of benazepril 20 mg and amlodipine 5 mg daily (the dosage of ACE inhibitor could be doubled after one month when necessary, and the dosage of diuretic and calcium channel blocker could be doubled after 2 months) *vs* the combination of benazepril 20 mg and hydrochlorothiazide 12.5 mg daily, induced a more marked reduction of SBP (129.3 mmHg *vs* 130 mmHg; p = 0.05), increased the percentage of patients in whom BP was controlled (< 140/90 mmHg) (81.7% *vs* 78.5%; p < 0.001) and decreased by 19,6% (p < 0.001) the risk of developing one of the components of the primary composite endpoint comprising cardiovascular mortality, nonfatal stroke and myocardial infarction, hospitalization for unstable angina, coronary revascularization and resuscitated sudden death. For the secondary endpoint of death from cardiovascular causes, nonfatal myocardial infarction and stroke, the hazard ratio was 0.79 (p = 0.002).

■ In the absence of left ventricular dysfunction and/or heart failure, the combination of an ARB and an ACE inhibitor does not improve the efficacy of the ACE inhibitor in terms of cardiovascular risk prevention, but is associated with a higher risk of hypotension and renal impairment.

■ In the **ONTARGET** study (see p. 25), addition of the combination of telmisartan 80 mg- ramipril 10 mg daily *vs* addition of ramipril 10 mg daily did not reduce the incidence of the cardiovascular events of the primary composite endpoint observed in 16.46% *vs* 16.3% of cases (RR: 0.99 [0.92-1.07]), or the incidence of the events of the secondary endpoint (cardiovascular mortality, myocardial infarction, stroke) observed in 14.11% *vs* 14.1% of cases (RR: 1.0 [0.93-1.09]), but increased the risk of hypotension by a factor of 2.75 ($p < 0.00001$), the risk of syncope by a factor of 1.95 ($p < 0.032$) and the risk of renal impairment by a factor of 1.58 ($p = 0.005$).

Addition of statins

■ In hypertensive patients with high cardiovascular risk, a statin should be added to antihypertensive therapy, regardless of the baseline total cholesterol (see p. 28, 43).

Addition of aspirin

■ In primary prevention, systematic addition of low-dose aspirin to antihypertensive therapy is not recommended, as its beneficial effect is counterbalanced by the increased bleeding risk.

■ In the **HOT** study conducted in 18,790 hypertensive patients (DBP: 110-115 mmHg) with a mean follow-up of 3.8 years, addition of aspirin 75 mg daily *vs* placebo to antihypertensive therapy decreased the incidence of major cardiovascular events by 15% ($p = 0.03$) and myocardial infarction by 36% ($p = 0.003$), without reducing the stroke rate, but this beneficial effect was counterbalanced by an almost twofold higher risk of nonfatal major bleeding (RR: 1.8; $p < 0.001$).

■ In contrast, in secondary prevention, low-dose aspirin (75 mg/day) must be systematically added to antihypertensive therapy.

■ A platelet aggregation inhibitor must be an integral part of the treatment prescribed after acute coronary syndrome or myocardial infarction, especially when treated by stenting, stroke or arterial disease of the lower limbs. In most cases, it is associated with a beta-blocker, a statin and an ACE inhibitor or ARB.

■ A platelet aggregation inhibitor should only be prescribed when HT has been controlled by treatment and in the absence of contraindications to the use of this class.

HT and LVH

■ HT is often accompanied by left ventricular hypertrophy (LVH), which has now been demonstrated to have a harmful role.

■ The frequency of LVH varies as a function of the severity of HT. The frequency of LVH evaluated by echocardiography is 15-20% in mild HT and 50% in severe HT (*N Engl J Med* 1990; *322*: 1561-1566).

■ Increased left ventricular mass alters cardiac functioning.

■ It increases the incidence of atrial and ventricular arrhythmias, increases myocardial ischemia and decreases left ventricular relaxation and compliance.

■ Increased left ventricular mass is an independent cardiovascular risk factor.

■ In the study by **Levy** conducted in 3,220 subjects included in the **Framingham** study, with a follow-up of 4 years, the presence of LVH detected by echocardiography doubled the risk of cardiovascular disease in patients of either sex and increased the risk of cardiovascular death by a factor of 5 in males and a factor of 3 in females.

■ Treatment of HT induces regression of LVH, as demonstrated to varying degrees with all classes of antihypertensives with the exception of minoxidil and hydralazine.

◆ *Regression of left ventricular mass during antihypertensive therapy appears to be partly independent of blood pressure reduction.*

■ This was demonstrated by the **LIFE** study (see p. 22) conducted in hypertensive patients with ECG signs of LVH in whom losartan 50-100 mg daily decreased LVH (p < 0.0001) to a greater extent than atenolol 50-100 mg daily, as reflected by reduction of the Cornell product and the Sokolow-Lyon index.

■ This was also demonstrated by an ancillary study of the **HOPE** study, in which ramipril 10 mg daily decreased left ventricular hypertrophy assessed on ECG.

■ This was also demonstrated by the **LIVE** study conducted in 411 hypertensive patients with LVH; with a follow-up of 48 weeks, for an equivalent degree of blood pressure reduction, indapamide SR 1.5 mg daily significantly decreased the left ventricular mass index (p < 0.001), while enalapril 20 mg daily had no effect on this parameter.

■ This was also demonstrated the **PICXEL** study, conducted in 556 hypertensive patients, in whom with a follow-up of one year, the combination of perindopril 2 mg daily and indapamide 0.625 mg daily *vs* enalapril 10 mg daily (possible doubling of the dosage on two occasions) decreased LVH to a significantly greater extent, especially when LVH was concentric (-13.6 *vs* -3.9 g/m^2; p < 0.001).

◆ *The clinical consequences of regression of left ventricular mass have not been evaluated by a large-scale clinical trial, but many data suggest that it could significantly reduce morbidity and mortality.*

HT and dyslipidemia

■ HT and dyslipidemia is a frequent and serious association.

■ In a study by **Perreault** conducted in 7,814 patients aged 35 to 74 years, free of cardiovascular disease, the total cholesterol/HDL-cholesterol ratio was higher in both male and female hypertensive subjects than in age-matched normotensive subjects.

■ In the Swedish study by **Sundström** initiated between 1970 and 1973 on a population of male hypertensive patients with a follow-up of 20 years, echocardiography performed in 475 subjects showed that the presence of dyslipidemia at the age of 50 significantly increased the risk of developing LVH at the age of 70 from 27% to 41%.

■ In hypertensive patients with a high cardiovascular risk (10-year risk of a cardiovascular event ≥ 20% according to the **Framingham** equation or ≥ 5% risk of death according to the **SCORE** grid), it is recommended to add a statin to antihypertensive therapy because statins significantly decrease this risk, especially the risk of stroke, regardless of baseline total cholesterol.

◆ *This was demonstrated in high-risk hypercholesterolemic hypertensive patients.*

■ In the **ASCOT-LLA** study, the lipid-lowering treatment arm of the double-blind ASCOT study conducted with a 2 x 2 factorial plan in 19,342 hypertensive patients, with a mean follow-up of 3.3 years, the addition of atorvastatin 10 mg daily *vs* placebo to antihypertensive therapy, when total cholesterol was ≥ 2.51 g/L (6.5 mmol/L), very significantly reduced the risk of the composite endpoint comprising nonfatal myocardial infarction and fatal coronary event by 36% (p = 0.0005) by the first year.

◆ *This was demonstrated in high-risk normocholesterolemic hypertensive patients.*

■ In the **HPS** study conducted in 20,636 patients of both sexes with a mean age of 40 years, a high cardiovascular risk (because of HT treated in men over the age of 70 years, history of myocardial infarction, unstable or stable angina, myocardial revascularization, non-hemorrhagic stroke or TIA, arterial disease of the lower limbs, insulin-dependent or non-insulin-dependent diabetes) and total cholesterol > 1.35 g/L (3.5 mmol/L), with a mean follow-up of 5.0 years, simvastatin 40 mg once daily *vs* placebo decreased total mortality due to a highly significant 18% reduction of coronary mortality (p = 0.0005) and reduced the risk of nonfatal myocardial infarction or coronary mortality (p < 0.0001), the risk of fatal or nonfatal stroke (p < 0.0001) and the coronary or non-coronary revascularization rate by about 25% (p < 0.0001).

■ Risk reduction was observed in all predefined subgroups, regardless of gender, age, baseline total cholesterol (< 1.93 g/L [5.0 mmol/L] or ≥ 2.32 g/L [6.0 mmol/L]) and LDL-cholesterol (< 1.16 g/L [3.0 mmol/L] or ≥ 1.35 g/L [3.5 mmol/L]).

◆ *Very surprisingly, this favorable effect was not observed in the* **ALLHAT-LLT** *study, but the results of this study do not invalidate the beneficial effect of statins, which has been extensively demonstrated.*

■ Moreover, meta-analysis including the patients of the **ALL-HAT-LLT** study with those of previous studies (a total of 64,736 patients) showed that statins decrease total cholesterol by about 20%, coronary events by 27% and mortality by 14%.

■ The target LDL-cholesterol level depends on the number of cardiovascular risk factors.

■ In primary prevention, the target LDL-C is < 1.6 g/L (4.1 mmol/L) when HT is associated with one other cardiovascular risk factor and < 1.3 g/L (2.6 mmol/L) when HT is associated with 2 other cardiovascular risk factors.

■ In secondary prevention (coronary heart disease or history of vascular disease, especially stroke), the target LDL-C must be ≤ 1.0 g/L (2.56 mmol/L).

HT of the elderly

■ HT of the elderly is now recognized as a distinct entity.

■ For a long time, HT of the elderly was neglected and/or not treated, as, up until a few years ago, HT of the elderly was considered to ensure effective perfusion of target organs threatened by decreased arterial elasticity. We now know that treatment of HT of the elderly is well tolerated and significantly improves the prognosis of the disease.

■ Isolated systolic HT constitutes the commonest form of hypertension in subjects over the age of 65.

◆ *According to the JNC-VI and **ISH/WHO** criteria, it is defined by a SBP ≥ 140 mmHg and a DBP ≤ 90 mmHg and comprises three grades: grade 1: SBP < 160 mmHg; grade 2: SBP < 180 mmHg; and grade 3: SBP ≥ 180 mmHg. An increased pulse pressure is one of the main determinants of cardiovascular risk in this situation.*

■ The positive diagnosis of isolated systolic HT of the elderly is now facilitated by self-measurement and ABPM, as the simple office measurement of blood pressure overestimates blood pressure in about 20% of cases.

■ In the **SHEAF** study, office blood pressure measurements overestimated blood pressure in 17% of cases compared to the figures obtained by self-measurement.

■ In the study by **Fagard** conducted in 695 of the 4,695 patients included in the **SYST-EUR** study, the mean of 6 office blood pressure measurements was 174 ± 11/86 ± 6 mmHg, while ABPM was normal (SBP < 140 mmHg between 10:00 a.m. and 8:00 p.m.) in 24% of patients, therefore questioning the validity of the diagnosis of isolated systolic HT.

■ More specifically in the elderly, treatment of HT reduces the cardiovascular risk and decreases the risk of dementia.

■ Furthermore, the absolute benefit of antihypertensive therapy is greater in the elderly than in young subjects, as the absolute cardiovascular risk increases with age.

■ Treatment of hypertension of the elderly, whether systolic-diastolic hypertension or isolated systolic hypertension, reduces the cardiovascular risk.

■ This was demonstrated by the **EWPHE, STOP-Hypertension-1, MRC-Older, CASTEL, STONE, STOP-Hypertension-2, SCOPE, ANBP 2, SHEP, SYST-Eur, and SYST-China** studies and was confirmed by 5 meta-analyses: those by **Mac Mahon and Rodgers, Insua, Mulrow, Pearce,** and **Gueyffier.**

■ Treatment of HT of the elderly, regardless of the type of HT, reduces the risk of dementia.

■ This was demonstrated by an ancillary study of the **SYST-EUR** study conducted in hypertensive patients over the age of 60 years with isolated systolic hypertension. With a mean follow-up of 2 years, antihypertensive therapy (nitrendipine 10-40 mg daily possibly associated with enalapril 5-20 mg daily and/or hydrochlorothiazide 12.5-25 mg daily) *vs* placebo decreased the incidence of dementia by 50%.

■ This was also demonstrated by analysis of patients of the **SCOPE** study, in whom the intellectual score assessed by MMSE was ≤ 28 but > 24. In these patients, who represented 42% of the total study population, candesartan therapy significantly (p = 0.04) decreased cognitive impairment *vs* the control group.

■ This was especially demonstrated by the **PROGRESS** study conducted in 6,105 patients (mean age: 64 years) with a history of stroke or ischemic TIA, 48% of whom were hypertensive; with a mean follow-up of 3.9 years, perindopril 4 mg daily, possibly associated with indapamide 2.5 mg daily, *vs* placebo tended to reduce the relative risk of dementia by 12% (p = 0.2; NS) and significantly (p = 0.01) decreased by 19% the risk of cognitive impairment, reflected by loss of at least 3 points on the MMSE.

■ Treatment of HT is fully justified after the age of 80 years, as it significantly decreases the cardiovascular risk.

■ Treatment of isolated systolic HT: the meta-analysis by **Gueyffier** based on data concerning 1,132 patients over the age of 80 years included in 5 trials, showed that, compared to the control group, antihypertensive therapy decreased the relative risk of fatal or nonfatal stroke by 34% (p = 0.014), that of major cardiovascular events by 22% (p = 0.01) and that of heart failure by 39% (p = 0.001). In contrast, mortality data were not conclusive.

■ In the case of systolo-diastolic hypertension and isolated systolic HT, this has been recently and unambiguously demonstrated by the **HYVET** study conducted in 3,845 hypertensive patients (SBP: 160-199 mmHg; DBP < 110 mmHg; mean: 172.0/90.8 mmHg) with a mean age of 83.5 years, 65% of whom were already receiving antihypertensive therapy; with a median follow-up of 1.8 year, the addition of indapamide SR 1.5 mg daily, possibly associated with perindopril 2-4 mg daily when the BP goal (150/80 mmHg) was not achieved, *vs* placebo, induced a supplementary lowering of BP by 15/6 mmHg, decreased the global incidence of stroke by 30% (p = 0.055) (primary endpoint); it also reduced mortality by 21% (p = 0.0019), and the incidence of fatal stroke by 39% (p = 0.046); it also reduced the incidence of heart failure by 64% (p < 0.0001) and the incidence of any cardiovascular event by 34% (p < 0.001) (secondary endpoints); but it did not modify the incidence of dementia, as demonstrated by the ancillary **HYVET-COG** study. The indapamide-perindopril combination was well tolerated and no statistically significant difference was observed between the 2 treatment arms for serum potassium, serum uric acid, serum creatinine and blood glucose. Furthermore, at the end of the study, 73.4% of patients assigned to active treatment received the indapamide-perindopril combination.

■ Treatment of HT of the elderly must comply with 3 essential rules: try to achieve SBP < 150 mmHg without inducing orthostatic hypotension; initiate treatment with low-dose monotherapy without sodium restriction; do not coprescribe more than 3 antihypertensive drugs.

HT and diabetes (see p. 63)

HT and coronary heart disease

■ After an acute coronary event, control of any HT reduces the recurrence rate and coronary mortality by 20%.

■ This was demonstrated by retrospective analysis of the subgroup of hypertensive patients included in the **AIRE** study.

■ Antihypertensive therapy is therefore beneficial in hypertensive patients with coronary heart disease and it is recommended to achieve a BP ≤ 130/80 mmHg by prescribing, as first-line treatment:

■ In hypertensive patients with stable coronary heart disease, a beta-blocker or long-acting calcium channel blocker.

■ In hypertensive patients post-myocardial infarction, a beta-blocker or ACE inhibitor.

■ In hypertensive patients with coronary heart disease, ramipril and perindopril are particularly effective, while verapamil can constitute an alternative to atenolol.

■ In the **HOPE** primary and secondary prevention study conducted in 9,297 patients with a mean age of 66 years and high cardiovascular risk (46.8% of subjects included were hypertensive), but not presenting either left ventricular dysfunction or heart failure, the addition of ramipril 10 mg daily *vs* placebo to standard therapy significantly decreased the relative risk of the main composite endpoint (myocardial infarction, stroke or cardiovascular mortality) by 22% (p < 0.001) and the relative risk of each component of this primary endpoint with a follow-up of 5 years.

■ In the **EUROPA** study conducted in 12,218 patients with coronary heart disease, 54.2% of whom were hypertensive, perindopril 8 mg once daily *vs* placebo in addition to standard therapy, with a mean follow-up of 4.2 years, reduced the relative risk of the main composite endpoint comprising cardiovascular death, non fatal myocardial infarction and resuscitated cardiac arrest by 20% (p = 0.0003) and the relative risk of non-fatal myocardial infarction by 22% (p = 0.001) and tended to reduce total mortality by 11%. This beneficial effect was observed regardless of the patient's risk level (i.e. in both sexes, regardless of age, in the presence or absence of a history of myocardial infarction, diabetes, HT, peripheral artery disease) and regardless of concomitant treatment (and especially, in the presence or absence of statins, beta-blockers).

■ In the **INVEST** study conducted in 22,576 hypertensive patients with coronary heart disease, with a mean follow-up of 2.7 years, verapamil SR 240 mg daily, possibly associated with trandolapril 2 mg daily, was found to be as effective as atenolol 50 mg daily, possibly associated with hydrochlorothiazide 25 mg daily, on blood pressure control and prevention of major cardiovascular events.

HT and stroke

■ After a stroke, BP control significantly reduces not only the risk of recurrence, but also the incidence of major cardiovascular events.

■ This was demonstrated by the **PROGRESS** double-blind study conducted in 6,105 hypertensive (48%) or normotensive (52%) patients with a history of TIA or stroke without major disabling sequelae during the previous 5 years. With a follow-up of 4 years, active treatment including, in addition to standard therapy, perindopril 4 mg daily, possibly associated with indapamide 2.5 mg daily *vs* placebo significantly reduced the risk of another stroke (primary endpoint) by 28% (p < 0.0001), the incidence of major cardiovascular events (vascular mortality, myocardial infarction and nonfatal stroke) by 26% (p < 0.001) and the incidence of dementia and cognitive disorders secondary to another stroke (secondary endpoints) by 34% and 45%, respectively.

◆ *According to the Task Force of the European Society of Cardiology (Eur Heart J 2004; 25:1454-1470), ACE inhibitors represent the first-line treatment for HT in patients with a history of myocardial infarction or stroke. This recommendation has not been questionned by PRoFESS results (see p. 187, 190).*

Assessment of blood pressure control

■ Blood pressure control of hypertensive patients is still very insufficient.

■ Unfortunately, the rule of halves launched in the USA in the 1960s still applies.

■ According to this rule, only 50% of hypertensive patients know they are hypertensive; only 50% of them are treated; and only 50% of treated patients (i.e. 25% of the initial population) have a normal blood pressure.

■ According to the **NHANES III** study, the percentage of hypertensive patients aged 18 to 74 years in whom HT is controlled is only 24.4% in the USA and the situation is no better in the rest of the world.

■ In France, the **PHARE 1** survey conducted in 1994/1995 by 235 general practitioners in 12,351 subjects showed that only 24% of treated hypertensive patients had a normal blood pressure; 5 years later, this rate had increased to 31.5% in the **PHARE 2** survey.

■ The control of isolated systolic HT is still very insufficient.

■ According to the **NHANES III** study, and contrary to a widely held belief, this type of HT is poorly controlled by treatment in 65% of cases, especially in the elderly.

■ The control of HT is far from satisfactory, even in secondary prevention.

■ This was demonstrated by the **EUROASPIRE I, EUROASPIRE II** and **EUROASPIRE III** studies conducted in Europe between 1995 and 2007 on 8,547 patients hospitalized for acute coronary syndrome and/or myocardial revascularization by coronary artery bypass graft or coronary angioplasty. The percentage of hypertensive subjects (SBP $\geq$ 140 mmHg and/or DBP $\geq$ 90 mmHg) has remained stable over time, at 54.6%, 54%, and 54.2%, respectively, and has therefore not improved.

■ It is therefore not surprising that male and female hypertensive patients currently have a higher risk of total and cardiovascular mortality than the normotensive population.

■ This had been already shown by the **Glasgow Blood Pressure Clinic** study.

■ It was also demonstrated by the **MPPT** study conducted in 7,495 male subjects; with a follow-up of 15 years, the 686 hypertensive patients initially aged 52 years, in whom blood pressure was controlled during treatment, presented a higher total mortality (37.4% *vs* 29.2%; p < 0.001) than 6,810 normotensive control subjects.

New BHS-NICE guidelines (June 2006)

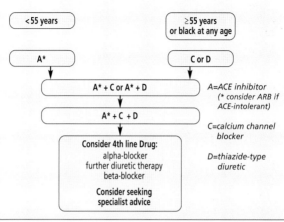

available at: http://www.nice.org.uk/page.aspx?o=cg34

JNC-VI classification* *(Arch Intern Med. 1997;157:2413-2446)*			
Blood pressure (mmHg)	**SBP**		**DBP**
Optimal	< 120	and	< 80
Normal	< 130	and	< 85
High-normal	130-139	or	85-89
Hypertension	**≥ 140**	**or**	**≥ 90**
• Stage 1	140-159	or	90-99
• Stage 2	160-179	or	100-109
• Stage 3	≥ 180	or	≥ 110
Isolated systolic hypertension	≥ 140	and	< 90

In diabetic patients, it is recommended to lower blood pressure to below 130-85 mmHg.

* This classification concerns adults over the age of 18.

Key messages of JNC-VII
(JAMA 2003;289:2560-2572)

- After the age of 50 years, SBP ≥140 mmHg is a much more important cardiovascular risk factor than DBP.

- The risk of cardiovascular disease starts at 115-75 mmHg and doubles with each increment of 20-10 mmHg.

- Individuals with a SBP of 120 to 139 mmHg or DBP of 80 to 89 mmHg should be considered as prehypertensive and require health-promoting lifestyle modifications to prevent cardiovascular disease.

- Thiazide diuretics should be used in drug treatment for most patients with uncomplicated hypertension. Certain high-risk conditions may require initial use of other antihypertensive drug classes (beta-blockers, calcium channel blockers, ACE inhibitors, angiotensin II receptor antagonists).

- Most patients with hypertension will require 2 or more antihypertensive medications to achieve goal BP (<140-90 mmHg, or <130-80 mmHg for patients with diabetes or chronic kidney disease).

- If initial BP is more than 20-10 mmHg above goal BP, consideration should be given to initiating therapy with 2 antihypertensive agents, including a thiazide diuretic.

- The most effective therapy prescribed by the most careful clinician will control hypertension only if patients are sufficiently motivated and the clinician plays an essential role on this aspect.

CHAPTER 2

Hypercholesterolemia

Factual data

■ The therapeutic management of dyslipidemic patients must integrate correction of all risk factors and is designed to delay the development (primary prevention) or recurrence (secondary prevention) of complications of atherosclerosis.

■ The benefit of cardiovascular prevention has been demonstrated in subjects aged 70 to 80 years, postmenopausal women, hypertensive patients, patients with type 2 diabetes and patients with a history of vascular disease.

■ Reduction of the cardiovascular risk is correlated with lowering of LDL-C, which is the best indicator of the efficacy of lipid-lowering treatment.

■ In patients with a high cardiovascular risk or in the context of secondary prevention, lipid-lowering drug treatment and the dose prescribed must comply with those demonstrated to be effective in the major clinical trials.

■ Standard practice is to start treatment as early as possible with a low dosage and to subsequently increase the dosage according to efficacy and safety.

■ The maximum efficacy of treatment is obtained in about 4 weeks.

■ Hypercholesterolemia increases the cardiovascular risk, but the intensity of management of hypercholesterolemia depends on the global vascular risk taking all associated risk factors into account.

■ For example, the combination of dyslipidemia and HT worsens the cardiovascular prognosis and must be treated energetically (see p. 30).

Non-pharmacological treatment

■ Diet is necessary but usually insufficient on its own, because, at best, it decreases LDL-C by only 10 to 15% and does not modify total mortality.

■ This was the conclusion of the meta-analysis by **Hooper** based on 27 studies comprising a total of 30,902 subjects, in whom dietary measures alone had no effect on total mortality, decreased cardiovascular events by 16% and tended to reduce cardiovascular mortality by 9%, with a follow-up of at least 2 years.

■ Dietary modification comprises 4 types of measures:

– reduction of dietary cholesterol, or consumption of foods enriched in plant sterols;

– reduction of the saturated fatty acid (animal fat);

– increased consumption of omega-3 polyunsaturated fatty acids (fish), as the meta-analysis by **Bucher** showed that such a diet reduced the risk of coronary events and stroke;

– increased consumption of fruit, vegetables and cereals.

Pharmacological treatment

Primary prevention

Statins

■ Statins reduce LDL-C by about 30% and decrease cardio-vascular morbidity and mortality.

◆ *This was demonstrated by the **WOSCOPS, AFCAPS/Tex-CAPS** and **HPS** studies.*

■ In the **WOSCOPS** study, which included 6,595 Scottish men with a mean LDL-C of 1.92 g/L (4.95 mmol/L) *vs* placebo, pravastatin 40 mg daily significantly decreased the incidence of coronary events by 31% (p < 0.001), cardiovascular mortality by 32% (p= 0.033) and total mortality by 22% (p = 0.051), with a mean follow-up of 4.9 years.

■ In the **AFCAPS/TexCAPS** study conducted in 6,605 subjects with a mean LDL-C of 1.50 g/L (3.87 mmol/L) *vs* placebo, lovastatin 20-40 mg daily decreased the risk of a major coronary events by 37% (p < 0.001) without modifying total mortality, with a mean follow-up of 5.2 years.

■ In the **HPS** primary and secondary prevention study conducted in 20,536 patients, simvastatin 40 mg daily significantly decreased all major vascular events by 24% (p < 0.0001), the risk of ischemic stroke by 27%, vascular mortality by 17% and total mortality by 12%, with a follow-up of 5 years.

■ Statins are the first-line treatment for pure or mixed hypercholesterolemia.

■ Ezetimibe, a new inhibitor of intestinal absorption of cholesterol, fibrates or nicotinic acid can be used as second-line therapy.

Fibrates

■ Prescription of fibrate monotherapy is reserved for particular cases.

■ According to the **NSFA** guidelines, this essentially concerns patients with severe isolated hypertriglyceridemia with serum triglycerides ≥ 4 g/L (4.56 mmol/L), and patients with low LDL-C (< 1 g/L, i.e. 2.58 mmol/L) and HDL-C (< 0.35 g/L, i.e. 0.9 mmol/L in males and < 0.40 g/L, i.e. 1.03 mmol/L in females) associated with serum triglycerides > 2.5 g/L (2.85 mmol/L).

■ A fibrate can also be used as second-line monotherapy for patients intolerant to statins.

■ If a fibrate administered at the usual dosage fails to achieve the target, it is not recommended to increase the prescribed dose, as it would provide only a limited additional benefit.

■ Colestyramine and gemfibrozil decrease LDL-C by 10 to 15% and reduce coronary morbidity and mortality.

■ This was demonstrated by the **LRC-CPPT** study conducted with colestyramine in 3,806 men and the **HHS** study conducted with gemfibrozil in 4,081 men.

■ In the meta-analysis by **Muldoon** based on 6 trials comprising 24,847 men, treatment reduced coronary mortality by 14.4% (p = 0.04) without significantly modifying total mortality.

■ Ezetimibe coprescribed with a statin ensures an additional reduction of LDL-C by as much as 25%.

■ This was demonstrated by the study by **Ballantyne** and the **EASE** study.

Secondary prevention

Statins

■ Statins significantly decrease cardiovascular morbidity and mortality and total mortality.

◆ *This was demonstrated by the 4S, CARE, LIPID and HPS studies.*

■ In the **4S** study, which included 4,444 patients with coronary heart disease with total cholesterol between 2.1 and 3.1 g/L (5.4 and 8 mmol/L), simvastatin 20-40 mg daily *vs* placebo decreased coronary mortality by 42% (RR 0.58 [0.46-0.73]), cardiovascular mortality by 35% and total mortality by 30%, with a mean follow-up of 5.4 years.

■ In the **CARE** study conducted in 4,159 patients with a history of myocardial infarction and LDL-C between 1.15 and 1.74 g/L (2.9 and 4.4 mmol/L), pravastatin 40 mg daily vs placebo decreased the risk of coronary mortality or myocardial infarction by 24% (p = 0.003) and tended to decrease total mortality of 9%, with a mean follow-up of 5 years.

■ In the **LIPID** study, which included 9,014 patients with coronary heart disease and total cholesterol between 1.55 and 2.71 g/L (4 and 7 mmol/L), pravastatin 40 mg daily vs placebo decreased coronary mortality by 24% (p < 0.0001), the risk of myocardial infarction by 29% (p < 0.001), and total mortality by 22% (p < 0.001), with a mean follow-up of 6.1 years.

■ In the **HPS** study conducted in 20,536 patients in a context of secondary prevention (documented ischemic heart disease, history of ischemic stroke, arterial disease of the lower limbs) and primary prevention in high-risk subjects (diabetes or hypertension in men over the age of 70), simvastatin 40 mg daily vs placebo significantly decreased the risk of all major vascular events by 24%, stroke by 27%, vascular mortality by 17% and total mortality by 12%, with a mean follow-up of 5 years.

◆ *The target LDL-C level in secondary prevention is ≤ 1 g/L (2.6 mmol/L).*

■ The beneficial effect of statins is obtained regardless of gender, age and especially baseline serum cholesterol.

■ The absence of difference between males and females was demonstrated in the **HPS** and **LIPID** studies.

■ The impact of statins on morbidity and mortality was identical in subjects over the age of 75 years and in younger patients in the **HPS** study. This was confirmed by the **PROSPER** study, which included 5,804 patients aged 70 to 82 years with a history of coronary heart disease or presenting a risk factor including diabetes, HT, and smoking with a mean LDL-C of 1.47 g/L. In this study, pravastatin 40 mg daily vs placebo significantly decreased the risk of death, myocardial infarction or stroke by 15%, with a mean follow-up of 3.2 years.

■ The beneficial effect is acquired regardless of the baseline total cholesterol and LDL-C levels, as demonstrated by the **4S, LIPID, CARE** and especially the **HPS** studies. In this last study, the reduction of morbidity and mortality with simvastatin was observed even in patients with normal serum cholesterol, supporting the pleiotropic effect of statins, independent of lowering of serum cholesterol.

◆ *Statins can therefore be safely used to decrease the 5-year risk of major cardiovascular events (coronary accident, coronary revascularization, stroke) by 1/5 per mmol/L of reduction of LDL-C.*

■ This was demonstrated by the **CTT** prospective meta-analysis of 14 randomized trials comprising a total of 90,056 subjects.

■ The absolute benefit is essentially correlated with the risk level of the subject concerned and the absolute reduction of LDL-C.

■ The use of high dose statins results is an almost linear relationship between reduction of cardiovascular risk and degree of lowering of LDL-C.

◆ *This was demonstrated, in the context of acute coronary syndromes, by the MIRACL and PROVE-IT studies, but the A-to-Z study did not reach the same conclusions.*

■ In the **MIRACL** study, conducted in 3,086 patients hospitalized for acute coronary syndrome without persistent ST-segment elevation, atorvastatin 80 mg daily, started 24 to 96 hours after admission significantly decreased the mean LDL-C level from 1.24 g/L (3.20 mmol/L) at baseline to 0.72 g/L (1.85 mmol/L) and significantly decreased the combined incidence of death, non-fatal myocardial infarction, resuscitated cardiac arrest or severe recurrent myocardial ischemia at the 16th week (14.8% *vs* 17.4%; p = 0.048); this difference was exclusively due to reduction of severe recurrent angina.

■ In the **PROVE-IT** study conducted in 4,162 patients with recent acute coronary syndrome (< 10 days), with total cholesterol ≤ 2,4 g/L (6,19 mmol/L) (median LDL-C: 1,06 g/L i.e. 2,73 mmol/L), atorvastatin 80 mg daily was more effective than pravastatin

40 mg daily to lower LDL-C on the 30th day from the baseline value of 1.3 g/L (3.35 mmol/L) in the two groups to 0.62 vs 0.95 g/L (1.60 vs 2.45 mmol/L). With a follow-up of 2 years, atorvastatin 80 mg daily reduced the composite endpoint, comprising total mortality, myocardial infarction, acute coronary syndrome, myocardial revascularization and stroke, by 16% (p = 0.005). The benefit was apparent by the 30th day. In terms of safety, atorvastatin 80 mg was associated with a threefold higher elevation of hepatic transaminases.

■ In the **A-to-Z** study conducted in 4,497 patients hospitalized for acute coronary syndrome, with a follow-up of 2 years, simvastatin 40 mg daily for the first month then 80 mg daily vs placebo for 4 months then replaced by simvastatin 20 mg daily, tended to decrease the risk of death, myocardial infarction and recurrence of acute coronary syndrome or stroke (14.4% vs 16.7%; p = 0.14; NS).

■ The meta-analysis by **Murphy** (see p. 101) of the PROVE-IT and A-to-Z studies recommended the use of high doses of statins.

◆ *This was demonstrated, in the context of chronic coronary insufficiency, by the **ALLIANCE**, **TNT**, and **IDEAL** studies.*

■ In the **ALLIANCE** study conducted in 2,442 patients with stable coronary heart disease, aggressive treatment by atorvastatin titrated to lower LDL-C to below 0.8 g/L (2.06 mmol/L) vs conventional management, decreased the incidence of major cardiac events by 17% (p = 0.02) with a follow-up of 4 years.

■ In the **TNT** study conducted in 10,001 patients with stable coronary heart disease, atorvastatin 80 mg daily vs atorvastatin 10 mg daily more markedly lowered LDL-C (0.77 vs 1.01 g/L [1.98 vs 2.60 mmol/L]) and, with a mean follow-up of 4.9 years, decreased the combined incidence of coronary mortality, non-fatal myocardial infarction, resuscitated cardiac arrest or stroke by 22% (p < 0.001) without modifying total mortality, but with an excess elevation of hepatic transaminases (1,2% vs 0,2% ; p < 0.001).

■ In the **IDEAL** study conducted in 8,888 patients ≤ 80 years of age with stable coronary heart disease and a history of myocardial infarction, high-dose atorvastatin 80 mg daily *vs* conventional-dose simvastatin 20 mg daily only tended to decrease the combined incidence of coronary mortality, nonfatal myocardial infarction, and resuscitated cardiac arrest (9.3% *vs* 10.4%; p = 0.07; NS) but significantly reduced the risk of nonfatal myocardial infarction (6.0% *vs* 7.2%; p = 0.02) and all major cardiovascular (p = 0.02) and coronary events (p < 0.001).

■ All of these trials, representing a total follow-up of 100,000 patient-years, showed that intensive treatment with high-dose statins significantly decreased the number of cardiovascular events and especially decreased coronary mortality and myocardial infarction by 16% (p = 0.0001).

◆ *This was demonstrated, in the context of stroke, by the SPARCL study.*

■ In the **SPARCL** study conducted in 4,731 patients free of coronary heart disease, but with a history of stroke or TIA during the 6 months preceding inclusion and with LDL-C between 1.0 and 1.9 g/L (2.6 to 4.9 mmol/L), addition of atorvastatin 80 mg daily *vs* placebo to standard therapy significantly lowered LDL-C (to 0.73 g/L [1.9 mmol/L] *vs* 1.29 g/L [3.3 mmol/L] with placebo) and decreased the incidence of fatal or nonfatal stroke by 16% (p = 0.05) with a mean follow-up of 4.9 years. Furthermore, although patients included in the study were free of any known coronary heart disease, intensive treatment with atorvastatin 80 mg daily decreased the incidence of major coronary events (cardiac mortality, myocardial infarction, resuscitated cardiac arrest) by 35% (p = 0.002) and the incidence of major coronary events and stroke by 20% (p = 0.002), but without modifying total mortality.

– This result was obtained at the price of a slight and non-significant increase (5%) of the hemorrhagic stroke rate (55 cases with atorvastatin 80 mg daily *vs* 33 with placebo, with no difference between the 2 groups in terms of fatal hemorrhagic stroke).

■ Similar findings were reported in the meta-analysis by **Amarenco**.

– In practice, this risk must be taken into account before administering high-dose statins to a patient with a history of hemorrhagic stroke.

■ The linear relationship between lowering of LDL-C and decreased cardiovascular risk persists at least until an LDL-C level of 0.70 g/L (1.80 mmol/L).

■ This was demonstrated, in particular, by the **TNT** and **IDEAL** studies.

■ The marked reduction of LDL-C obtained with high-dose statins slows progression of atheromatous plaque.

■ In the **REVERSAL** study conducted in 502 patients with coronary plaques demonstrated by intracoronary ultrasound, high-dose atorvastatin 80 mg daily *vs* pravastatin 40 mg daily lowered baseline LDL-C from 1.5 g/L (3.87 mmol/L) to 0.79 g/L (2.03 mmol/L) (*vs* 1.1 g/L [2.83 mmol/L] with pravastatin) and stabilized the course of intracoronary atheromatous plaque (non-significant 0.4% volume reduction *vs* 2.7% progression with pravastatin, [p = 0.02]), with a follow-up of 18 months.

■ In the **ASTEROID** study conducted in 507 patients, high-dose rosuvastatin 40 mg daily lowered LDL-C by 53.2% (p < 0.001) from 1.3 to 0.6 g/L (3.35 to 1.54 mmol/L), significantly increased HDL-C by 15% and decreased the volume of coronary atheroma assessed by intracoronary ultrasound by 6.8%, with a follow-up of 2 years.

■ In the **METEOR** study conducted in 984 middle-aged patients at low cardiovascular risk and presenting moderate, subclinical carotid atherosclerosis, high-dose rosuvastatin 40 mg daily *vs* placebo lowered LDL-C by 49% from 1.55 to 0.75 g/L (4.0 to 1.55 mmol/L), significantly increased HDL-C by 8% and significantly slowed progression of carotid intima-media thickness assessed by B-mode ultrasound, with a follow-up of 2 years.

■ High dosages of statins are generally well tolerated.

■ In the retrospective analysis by **Newman** based on 49 trials comprising 14,236 patients, treated for 2 weeks to 52 months, the adverse event rate was similar with atorvastatin 80 mg daily and atorvastatin 10 mg daily.

■ The meta-analysis by **Silva** reached the same conclusions (see p. 102).

■ If the target LDL-C is not achieved despite the maximum tolerated dose of statins, the addition of ezetimibe, a specific inhibitor of cholesterol absorption, may help to achieve this target.

■ In some cases, and with close surveillance of adverse events, a statin can be coprescribed with a fibrate or nicotinic acid.

Fibrates

■ In secondary prevention, the beneficial effect of fibrates on cardiovascular morbidity and mortality remains uncertain, as two studies have reported contradictory results.

■ In the **VA-HIT** study, which included 2,531 men with coronary heart disease and a low HDL-C ($\leq$ 0.40 g/L ie 1.03 mmol/L) and essentially normal LDL-C (mean: 1.12 g/L ie 2.89 mmol/L) with a mean serum triglycerides of 1.6 g/L ie 1.82 mmol/L, gemfibrozil 1200 mg daily vs placebo decreased the risk of coronary mortality or nonfatal myocardial infarction by 22% (p = 0.006) with a mean follow-up of 5.1 years.

■ However, in the **BIP** study conducted in 3,090 patients with coronary heart disease and HDL-cholesterol $\leq$ 0.45 g/L (1.16 mmol/L), LDL-C $\leq$ 1.80 g/L (4.64 mmol/L) and triglycerides $\leq$ 3 g/L (3.42 mmol/L), bezafibrate 400 mg daily vs placebo did not significantly decrease the combined risk of myocardial infarction and sudden death, with a mean follow-up of 6.2 years.

Dyslipidemia and HT (see p. 30)

Dyslipidemia and diabetes (see p. 69)

Conversion factors

Cholesterol	Glucose	Triglycerides
mmol/L x 0.387 = g/L	mmol/L x 0.18 = g/L	mmol/L x 0.875 = g/L
g/L x 2.58 = mmol/L	g/L x 5.55 = mmol/L	g/L x 1.14 = mmol/L

Calculation of LDL-C according to Friedewald's formula*

$$\text{LDL-C} = \text{total cholesterol} - \text{HDL-C} - \frac{\text{triglycerides}}{5}$$

* The parameters of the formula are expressed in g/L. This formula is only valid for serum triglycerides < 3 or 4 g/L (3.42 or 4.56 mmol/L).

Body Mass Index

$$\text{Body Mass Index} = \frac{\text{weight (kg)}}{\text{height (m)}^2}$$

International Obesity Task Force classification
(in: *Diab Metab* 1988;24 *[suppl 2]*:10-4)

• Normal	20-24
• Overweight	25-29
• Obesity	≥ 30
. moderate	30-34,9
. severe	35-39,9
. massive	≥ 40

When should lifestyle and diet
be modified?

Patient with high cardiovascular risk:
- Documented history of cardiovascular
  disease
- High-risk type 2 diabetes**
- Risk of development of a coronary
  event within 10 years ≥ 20%

≥ 3 risk factors*

LDL-C < 1.0 g/L
2.6 mmol/L

LDL-C < 1.3 g/L
3.35 mmol/L

*Cardiovascular risk factors used to estimate global cardiovascular risk.

- **Age**
  - Males ≥ 50 years.
  - Females ≥ 60 years.
- **Family history of early coronary disease**
  - Myocardial infarction or sudden death before the age of 55 in
    the father or 1st degree male relative.
  - Myocardial infarction or sudden death before the age of 65 in
    the mother or 1st degree female relative.
  - early stroke before the age of 45.
- **Current smoking** or stopped for less than 3 years.
- **Treated or untreated permanent hypertension**
- **Treated or untreated type 2 diabetes**
- **LDL-C ≥ 1.60 g/L (4.1 mmol/L)** regardless of gender
- **HDL-C < 0.40 g/L (1.0 mmol/L)** regardless of gender

Protective factor
- **HDL-C ≥ 0.60 g/L (1.5 mmol/L):** subtract "one risk" from risk level
  score.

f dyslipidemic patients
/w.afssaps.sante.fr)

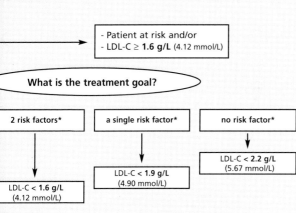

- Patient at risk and/or
- LDL-C ≥ **1.6 g/L** (4.12 mmol/L)

What is the treatment goal?

| 2 risk factors* | a single risk factor* | no risk factor* |

LDL-C < **2.2 g/L**
(5.67 mmol/L)

LDL-C < **1.9 g/L**
(4.90 mmol/L)

LDL-C < **1.6 g/L**
(4.12 mmol/L)

** High-risk type 2 diabetes
- Renal impairment,
- or at least two of the following risk factors: age, family history of early coronary disease, smoking, hypertension, HDL-C < 0.40 g/L (1.0 mmol/L), microalbuminuria (> 30 mg/24h).

Pleiotropic effects of statins

Definition

This term (*Curr Opin Lipidol* 1999;*10*:543-559) has been used to describe the poorly defined and non-quantified effects of statins, in addition to lowering of plasma LDL-C resulting from selective inhibition of HMG-CoA reductase.

Demonstration

- The existence of these pleiotropic effects is suggested by 2 findings:
  - The effect of statins is observed in normocholesterolemic patients as well as hypercholesterolemic patients.
  - In many studies of regression of atherosclerosis in response to statins, a clinical benefit is rapidly obtained even when anatomical lesions have regressed by only a few hundredths of a millimeter.
- It is not yet known whether the pleiotropic effects of statins alone, i.e. apart from a reduction of LDL-C, can induce a reduction of coronary events.

Description

- Stabilization of the atheromatous plaque.
  - Statins appear to act on macrophages which accumulate in the intima after having bound oxidized LDL; they decrease the LDL-C content of the lipid core, thereby preventing fissuring and rupture of the plaque; they appear to decrease the quantity of oxidized LDL (antioxidant action) in the plaque; they also appear to act on proliferation of smooth muscle cells of the plaque.
- Inhibition of platelet aggregation via inhibition of thromboxane A2.
- Action on coagulation by reduction of tPA activator or inhibition of the tissue factor.
- Inhibition of graft rejection in the case of heart transplantation and renal transplantation.
- Favorable action on blood pressure and osteoporosis.
- Improvement of endothelial function and restoration of nitric oxide (NO) production.
- Reduction of inflammatory phenomena documented by a decrease CRP levels.
- Development of neoangiogenesis.
- Antiarrhythmic effect.

CHAPTER 3

Diabetes

Factual data

■ The incidence of diabetes is regularly increasing as a result of the dramatic increase of obesity and sedentary lifestyle.

■ In 2025, the number of adult diabetics worldwide will reach 300 million (*vs* 135 million in 1995) and it has been estimated that the incidence of diabetes is going to increase by about 40% in industrialized countries and 170% in developing countries with a peak increase in India and China.

■ Diabetes currently affects 10.2 million Americans and an estimated 5.4 million elderly Americans suffer from undiagnosed diabetes. Type 2 diabetes accounts for more than 95% of all cases of diabetes and now affects children and adolescents.

■ Diabetes is a major cardiovascular risk factor in both sexes, but to a much greater extent in females than in males.

■ Diabetes multiplies the cardiovascular risk by 2 to 3 in males and by 3 to 5 in females.

■ Cardiovascular deaths represent 70% of all deaths of diabetic patients.

■ The cardiovascular risk increases with elevation of blood glucose, even well below the limits defining diabetes.

■ In the meta-analysis by **Coutinho** based on 95,783 subjects (94% men) with a mean follow-up of 12.4 years, the relative risk of a cardiovascular event was multiplied by 1.63 in subjects with a blood glucose of 1.10 g/L (6.1 mmol/L) *vs* those with blood glucose of 0.75 g/L (4.2 mmol/L).

■ Diabetes is often associated with other cardiovascular risk factors, mostly potentially modifiable, which worsen the prognosis.

■ In the **UKPDS 23** study conducted in 3,055 patients with a mean age of 52 years with recently diagnosed type 2 diabetes, the risk of developing coronary disease was multiplied by 1.5 to 2 in the presence of associated dyslipidemia, HT or smoking, with a mean follow-up of 7.9 years.

Definitions and diagnosis

■ Diabetes is strictly defined by the American Diabetes Association (ADA).

■ Diabetes is defined by fasting blood glucose $\geq$ 1.26 g/L (7.0 mmol/L) on two occasions and/or blood glucose $\geq$ 2 g/L, 2 hours after a 75 g oral glucose load, a simplified version of the now obsolete oral glucose tolerance test.

■ Impaired glucose tolerance is also precisely defined by the ADA.

■ Impaired glucose tolerance is defined by fasting blood glucose between 1.10 and 1.25 g/L (6.0 and 6.9 mmol/L) and/or blood glucose > 1.40 g/L (7.77 mmol/L) and < 2 g/L (11.1 mmol/L), 2 hours after a 75 g oral glucose load.

■ Early diagnosis of diabetes, before the onset of clinical symptoms and signs, is ideally based on a 75 gram oral glucose load with blood glucose assay while fasting and 2 hours after the glucose load.

■ A 75 g oral glucose load allows the early diagnosis of diabetes.

■ In the **DECODE** study, one third of the thousands of subjects evaluated would have been considered to be non-diabetic exclusively on the basis of fasting blood glucose assays.

■ Postprandial blood glucose assay cannot replace the 75 gram oral glucose load.

■ Although postprandial elevation of blood glucose is probably the earliest abnormality of blood glucose dysregulation, it cannot constitute a diagnostic test for two reasons: meals composed of carbohydrates, lipids and proteins are difficult to standardize and are not absorbed with the same reproducibility as an oral glucose load; and postprandial blood glucose has also been shown to be less discriminant than the 75 gram oral glucose load.

■ The glycosylated hemoglobin (HbA1c) level is not considered to be a diagnostic criterion of diabetes.

■ According to the WHO, HbA1c, which reflects the sum of circadian variations of blood glucose over the previous 6 to 8 weeks (corresponding to the life span of red blood cells (*Diabetes Care* 1982; *5*: 592-599), is not sufficiently precise, sensitive and reproducible.

■ However, HbA1c remains one of the essential parameters of the follow-up of diabetic patients.

Cardiovascular risk reduction

■ Cardiovascular risk reduction, whether primary or secondary, is based on a combination of clearly defined parameters.

Lifestyle modification

■ Patient education in order to adopt a healthier lifestyle improves metabolic control.

■ Every effort must be made to achieve smoking cessation, weight reduction based on a reduction of the caloric intake (decreased to about 1,500 kcal/day, fats must not exceed 30 to

35% of the caloric intake), increase dietary fibre intake (30 g/day), limited consumption of carbohydrates, regular exercise (at least 30 minutes a day, at least 5 days a week).

■ In the **UKPDS 7** study conducted in a population of patients with type 2 diabetes, a 5 kg weight loss lowered HbA1c by about 7% to an absolute value of about 7%.

Strict blood glucose control

■ Strict blood glucose control in diabetic patients designed to achieve HbA1c close to 6.5% compared to a less rigorous control significantly decreases the risk of microvascular (**UKPDS 33** and **34** studies) and macrovascular (**DCCT** and **EDIC** studies) complications and neuropathy.

■ In the **UKPDS 33** study conducted in 3,687 patients with type 2 diabetes (mean age 54 years), with a follow-up of 10 years, intensive treatment of diabetes (target blood glucose < 1.10 g/L [6.1 mmol/L]) reduced the risk of microvascular complications by 25% (p = 0.0099), but had no effect on the risk of macrovascular complications, especially myocardial infarction or sudden death.

■ The **UKPDS 34** study reported similar findings: with a follow-up of 9 years, strict blood glucose control did not modify the incidence of stroke.

■ However, in contrast, the **EDIC** study, which extended by 10 years the follow-up of the **DCCT** study conducted in patients with type 1 diabetes, intensified insulin therapy designed to achieve a mean HbA1c close to 7% for the first 7 to 10 years, compared to standard therapy, reduced the incidence of the composite endpoint comprising cardiovascular death, nonfatal myocardial infarction and stroke by 57% (p = 0.02) and each of the other components of cardiovascular risk by 42%.

■ Similarly the 10 year follow-up of **UKPDS** demonstrated that despite an early loss of glycemic differences between the conventional therapy (dietary restriction) or intensive therapy (either sulfonylurea or insulin or, in overweight patients, metformin) groups, a continued 24% (p = 0.01) reduction in microvascular disease, as well as a 15% (p = 0.01) risk reduction for myocardial infarction and a 13% (p = 0.007) risk reduction for death from any cause were observed in the intensive therapy group.

■The recent **ADVANCE, ACCORD** and **VADT** studies reached opposite conclusions as to the beneficial effect of strict blood glucose control on the risk of large-vessel disease but, like the **UKPDS 33** study, emphasized the fact that it significantly increased the incidence of severe hypoglycemia, which however remained low.

■The **ADVANCE** study, the only truly representative study of the global population, conducted in 11,140 patients with type 2 diabetes, with a mean age 66 ± 6 years and a median follow-up of 5 years, showed that a stricter blood glucose control based on gliclazide 30 to 120 mg once daily on top of other hypoglycemic drugs including insulin in 40.5% of cases (*vs* 24.1%) in order to lower HbA1c to ≤ 6.5%, *vs* standard blood glucose control, decreased the relative risk of developing the primary composite endpoint comprising major macrovascular events (cardiovascular mortality, myocardial infarction and nonfatal stroke) and microvascular events (onset or deterioration of nephropathy, retinopathy) by 10% (p = 0.01) and decreased the relative risk of microvascular events by 14% (p = 0.01) primarily because of a 21% reduction (p = 0.006) of the incidence of nephropathy. On the duration of the trial, strict blood glucose control did not reduce the incidence of major macrovascular events, especially cardiovascular mortality (p = 0.12) or all-cause mortality (p = 0.28). Although uncommon, acceptability showed a 2.7% rate of severe hypoglycemia *vs* 1.5% in the placebo group (p < 0.001). This event rate of severe hypoglycemia was around one quarter of that reported in the UKPDS 33 and one seventh of that observed in the ACCORD trial.

■In the **ADVANCE** study, joint effects of routine BP lowering (combination of perindopril and indapamide) and intensive glucose control (gliclazide MR-based) had fully additive effects and resulted annually in a 33% (p = 0.005) decrease of the rate of new or worsening nephropathy, a 18% (p = 0.04) decrease of all cause mortality and a 24% (p = 0.04) decrease in cardiovascular death.

■In the **ACCORD** study conducted in 10,251 patients with type 2 diabetes with a mean age of 62.2 years and a mean HbA1c of 8.1%, 35% of whom had a history of cardiovascular disease, with a mean follow-up of 3.5 years, intensive therapy (target HbA1c < 6.0%) using insulin in 67.3% of cases (*vs* 55.4%) *vs* standard therapy designed to achieve HbA1c between 7.0 and

7.9% did not significantly reduce the incidence of the primary composite endpoint comprising cardiovascular mortality, myocardial infarction and nonfatal stroke, but increased the mortality rate by a factor of 1.22 (p = 0.04), leading to discontinuation of the study. Intensive therapy was also more frequently accompanied by severe hypoglycemia requiring medical intervention (10.5% of cases *vs* 3.5%; p < 0.001) and weight gain > 10 kg compared to baseline (27.8% of cases *vs* 14.1%; p < 0.001).

■ In the **VADT** study conducted in 1,791 patients with type 2 diabetes, 97% males, with a mean age of 60 years on inclusion, no longer controlled by monotherapy alone and with a history of cardiovascular disease in 40% of cases; stricter blood glucose control designed to correct HbA1c (HbA1c < 7%) (by intensification of the dosages of the drugs which were the same in the 2 arms) *vs* standard blood glucose control (target HbA1c: 8 to 9%), with a follow-up of 7 years, only tended (NS) to reduce the incidence of the primary composite endpoint comprising cardiovascular mortality and major cardiovascular morbidity (myocardial infarction, stroke, heart failure, cardiac, cerebral or peripheral revascularization operations, amputations for acute ischemia of a lower limb) and did not significantly modify the incidence of its various components; in contrast, stricter blood glucose control significantly doubled the number of cases of severe hypoglycemia (HR: 2.062; p = 0.018).

■ These results can probably be explained by the particularly satisfactory control of the other risk factors which had already considerably reduced the cardiovascular risk of this diabetic population. These results do not invalidate the importance of good blood glucose control which ensures protection against the macrovascular risk, but suggest that treatment should be adapted to the patient's age and the history of diabetes while complying with international guidelines (in the **ACCORD** study, the target HbA1c set at less than 6% was much lower than that recommended in these guidelines).

Addition of other drugs to the treatment of diabetes

■ The addition of certain drugs to the basic treatment of diabetes reduces the cardiovascular risk.

Statins

■ It is now generally accepted that the addition of a statin to the treatment of diabetes must be considered in all patients with type 2 diabetes even in the absence of a history of cardiovascular disease, when total cholesterol is > 1.35 g/L (3.5 mmol/L) in order to lower total cholesterol by 30 to 40%.

■ In practice, a statin is almost systematically prescribed because this class of lipid-lowering agents has been shown to be the most powerful and the most effective to reduce LDL-C and cardiovascular risk.

Aspirin

■ In subjects with high cardiovascular risk, low-dose aspirin reduces the incidence of nonfatal coronary and/or cardiovascular events, but at the price of an increased bleeding risk.

■ This was demonstrated by the **TPT, HOT** and **PPP** studies.

■ In primary prevention, the prescription of low-dose aspirin remains controversial.

■ Some authors recommend systematic prescription of low-dose aspirin, while others consider that it is only required in the presence of at least 3 other major cardiovascular risk factors and/or microalbuminuria or especially proteinuria, as it is not devoid of long-term adverse effects.

■ In secondary prevention, when diabetes is associated with cardiovascular disease, the systematic addition of low-dose aspirin to standard therapy is recommended because it decreases the risk of cardiovascular events.

ACE inhibitors

■ When diabetes is associated with cardiovascular disease, the systematic addition of an ACE inhibitor (and low-dose aspirin) to standard therapy is recommended because it decreases the risk of cardiovascular events.

■ In the **MICRO-HOPE** study conducted in 3,577 diabetic patients included in the **HOPE** study, with a mean follow-up of 4.5 years, the addition of ramipril 10 mg vs placebo to standard therapy significantly decreased the main composite endpoint (myocardial infarction, stroke or cardiovascular mortality) by 25% (p = 0.0004) and significantly decreased the incidence of each of its components.

■ In the **PERSUADE** study conducted in the 1,502 diabetic patients of the **EUROPA** study (representing 12.3% of inclusions) with a mean follow-up of 4.3 years, addition of perindopril 8 mg once daily vs placebo to standard therapy tended to reduce the relative risk of the main composite endpoint comprising cardiovascular mortality, nonfatal myocardial infarction and resuscitated cardiac arrest by 19% (p = 0.13; NS).

■ In the **ADVANCE** study, systematic addition of a fixed combination of perindopril-indapamide to the standard therapy of patients with type 2 diabetes, whether they are hypertensive or normotensive, significantly reduces cardiovascular risk and the risk of total death.

■ Although ACE inhibitors and ARBs have a similar renal protective effect on diabetic nephropathy, ACE inhibitors may be the only class to prevent early mortality.

■ This was the conclusion of the meta-analysis by **Strippoli**, based on 43 trials comprising a total of 7,545 patients with various stages of diabetic nephropathy (from microalbuminuria to proteinuria), in whom ACE inhibitors vs placebo significantly reduced total mortality by 21% (RR: 0.79; 0.63-0.99), while ARBs did not modify total mortality. However, this result, derived from indirect comparison of these two therapeutic categories, using placebo as common comparator, needs to be confirmed.

■ In the **IDNT** and **RENAAL** studies conducted in respectively 1715 and 1513 hypertensive diabetics, active treatment (irbesartan and losartan, respectively) was not associated with a reduction of total mortality.

■ However, it must be remembered that, in 1,195 hypertensive diabetic patients with LVH on ECG included in the **LIFE** study, conducted in a total of 9,193 patients with a mean follow-up of 4.7 years, treatment with losartan 50-100 mg daily vs atenolol

50-100 mg daily reduced the relative risk of developing the primary endpoint comprising cardiovascular mortality, stroke or myocardial infarction by 24% (p = 0.031) and the risk of cardiovascular mortality by 37% (p = 0.028%).

Global management of cardiovascular risk factors

■ In patients with type 2 diabetes presenting micro-albuminuria, global management of all other cardiovascular risk factors reduces the incidence of macrovascular or microvascular events by about 50%.

■ In the randomized, open-label **Steno** study conducted in Denmark in 160 patients with type 2 diabetes (mean age: 55.1 years) presenting microalbuminuria, with a mean follow-up of 7.8 years, multifactorial management of cardiovascular risk *vs* conventional management significantly improved metabolic parameters and decreased the incidence of the main composite endpoint (cardiovascular mortality, nonfatal myocardial infarction, nonfatal stroke, myocardial revascularization procedure, amputation) by 53% (p = 0.008), nephropathy by 61%, retinopathy by 58% and autonomic neuropathy by 63%.

Diabetes and hypertension

■ Hypertension and diabetes are frequently associated, which increases the risks of atherosclerosis and cardiovascular disease.

■ This was demonstrated by the **MRFIT** and **PROCAM** studies.

■ According to **Sowers**, hypertension is 2 to 3 times more frequent in diabetic patients than in nondiabetic patients; hypertensive patients are also at greater risk of diabetes than normotensive subjects.

■ In diabetic hypertensive patients, strict blood pressure control significantly improves the cardiovascular prognosis compared to less strict blood pressure control.

■ In the 1,501 diabetic hypertensive patients included in the **HOT** study, the DBP ≤ 80 mmHg goal *vs* the DBP ≤ 90 mmHg goal was accompanied by a 51% reduction of major cardiovascular events (p = 0.05).

■ In the **UKPDS 38** study conducted in 1,148 hypertensive patients with type 2 diabetes, with a mean follow-up of 8.4 years, strict blood pressure control (BP goal < 150/85 mmHg) *vs* less strict blood pressure control lowered blood pressure to a significantly greater extent and reduced the relative risk of a diabetes-related complication by 24% (p = 0.0046).

■ In the **UKPDS 36** study conducted in 3,642 type 2 diabetic patients with a mean follow-up of 10.5 years, each 17 mmHg reduction of mean SBP decreased the risk of all diabetes-related complications by 12% (p < 0.0001) and the risk of myocardial infarction by 11% (p = 0.0001); the lowest risk was observed for SBP < 120 mmHg.

■ It is recommended to lower blood pressure to ≤ 130/80 mmHg in all diabetic hypertensive patients to ensure optimal cardiovascular risk prevention.

■ Adequate blood pressure control and detection of microalbuminuria reduce the morbidity related to microvascular and macrovascular complications.

■ The degree of blood pressure reduction achieved is more important than the choice of antihypertensive drug, but inhibition of the renin-angiotensin-aldosterone system may have an additional beneficial effect independently of blood pressure reduction *per se*.

■ Blood pressure control is therefore at least or even more effective than strict blood glucose control, but this blood pressure goal is difficult to achieve and often requires a combination of several antihypertensive drugs.

■ In principle, the five different classes of antihypertensive drugs can be used in hypertensive diabetics.

Diuretics and beta-blockers

■ However, diuretics and beta-blockers must be avoided as first-line treatment, although they have been shown to be effective as monotherapy, because they can exacerbate insulin resistance and lead to a higher dosage or an increased number or antidiabetic drugs (see **Messerli** p. 18). In subjects with impaired glucose tolerance, diuretics and beta-blockers can lead to the earlier prescription of more intensive antidiabetic therapy. This may not apply to new generation beta-blockers, carvedilol and nebivolol, which do not affect glucose metabolism and insulin sensitivity. Clear proofs are still awaited.

Calcium channel blockers

■ Calcium channel blockers are effective as demonstrated by the study on the subgroup of 492 hypertensive diabetic patients included in the **SYST-EUR** study; with a follow-up of 2 years, nitrendipine *vs* placebo decreased the relative risks of stroke by 73%, cardiovascular events by 69% (*vs* -25% [p = 0.01] in diabetic not patients of the study), 76% the cardiovascular mortality (*vs* -13% [p = 0.02] in nondiabetic patients of the study), and total mortality by 55% (*vs* -6% [p = 0.04] in nondiabetic patients of the study).

Angiotensin-converting enzyme (ACE) inhibitors and angiotensin II receptor blockers (ARBs)

■ Renin-angiotensin system inhibitors (ACE inhibitors or ARBs) ensure better renal protection and must be an integral part of treatment, especially in patients with micro-albuminuria; their prescription requires strict surveillance of renal function.

◆ *ACE inhibitors and ARBs have a nephroprotective effect independent of their favorable action on BP and have been shown to be superior to other drugs to prevent, delay or slow the progression of nephropathy.*

ACE inhibitors

■ In the **MICRO-HOPE** study conducted in 3,577 diabetic patients included in the **HOPE** study who also had either a history of cardiovascular disease or at least one other risk factor, in the absence of proteinuria on urinary dip-sticks, heart failure or left ventricular dysfunction, the addition of ramipril 10 mg *vs* placebo to standard therapy significantly decreased the incidence of frank nephropathy by 24% (p = 0.027), the main composite endpoint (myocardial infarction, stroke or cardiovascular mortality) by 25% (p = 0.0004) and each of its components by 22% to 37%, with a mean follow-up of 4.5 years.

■ In the **PREMIER** study conducted in 481 hypertensive patients with a mean age of 59 ± 9 years, with type 2 diabetes and microalbuminuria (> 20 and < 500 µg/min), with a follow-up of one year, the combination of perindopril 2 to 8 mg and indapamide 0.6 to 2.5 mg daily *vs* enalapril 10 to 40 mg daily significantly decreased SBP, DBP and urinary albumin excretion.

■ In the **NESTOR** study conducted in 570 hypertensive patients with a mean age 60.0 ± 9.9 years with type 2 diabetes and microalbuminuria (20-200 µg/min) and a follow-up of one year, treatment with indapamide SR 1.5 mg daily was as effective as treatment with enalapril 10 mg daily to control blood pressure and reduce microalbuminuria.

■ In the **ADVANCE** study, perindopril-indapamide fixed combination was associated with a significant 21% (p < 0.0001) reduction in all renal events, with a borderline significant 18% (p = 0.055) reduction in new or worsening nephropathy and a significant 21% (p < 0.0001) reduction in the development of microalbuminuria. Over 5 years, one patient in every 20 assigned active treatment would have avoided one renal event (mostly the onset of new microalbuminuria).

Angiotensin II receptor blockers (ARBs)

■ In the **IRMA II** study conducted in 590 hypertensive patients with a mean age of 58.4 ± 8 years, with type 2 diabetes, microalbuminuria (20 to 200 µg/min, i.e. 28.8 to 288 mg/24 h) and serum creatinine ≤ 15 mg/L (133 µmol/L) in men and ≤ 11 mg/L (97 µmol/L) in women, with a follow-up of 2 years, irbesartan

150 mg daily *vs* placebo decreased the risk of diabetic nephropathy by 39% (p = 0.08), while irbesartan 300 mg daily decreased this risk by 70% (p < 0.001).

■ In the **IDNT** study conducted in 1,715 hypertensive diabetic with a mean age of 59.3 ± 7.1 years presenting frank nephropathy (proteinuria ≥ 0.9 g/24 h and serum creatinine between 11 and 30 mg/L [97 and 265 μmol/L]), with a mean follow-up of 2.6 years, irbesartan 300 mg daily administered in addition to standard therapy *vs* amlodipine 10 mg daily and placebo reduced the primary endpoint, comprising doubling of serum creatinine, appearance of end-stage renal disease and all-cause mortality, by 20% *vs* placebo (p = 0.02) and 23% *vs* amlodipine (p = 0.006), with no difference in the blood pressure levels achieved with the 2 antihypertensives.

■ In the **RENAAL** study conducted in 1,513 hypertensive patients with a mean age of 59.6 years, with type 2 diabetes and frank nephropathy (24-hour proteinuria > 500 mg; serum creatinine ≥ 15-30 mg/L), with a mean follow-up of 3.5 years, the addition of losartan 50-100 mg daily *vs* placebo to the treatment of diabetes decreased the primary endpoint, comprising doubling of serum creatinine, end-stage renal disease or death, by 16% (p = 0.02), independently of the degree of blood pressure reduction. It also reduced the risk of progression to end-stage renal disease requiring hemodialysis or transplantation by 28% (p = 0.002), the risk of doubling of serum creatinine by 25% (p = 0.006) and increased proteinuria by 35% (p < 0.0001).

Combinations of ACE inhibitors and other antihypertensive drugs

■ ACE inhibitors may be successfully combined with other antihypertensive drugs.

■ In the **BENEDICT** study conducted in 1,204 hypertensive patients with type 2 diabetes, with a mean follow-up of 3.6 years, the combination of trandolapril 2 mg and verapamil SR 180 mg daily and trandolapril 2 mg daily administered alone *vs* placebo decreased the risk of nocturnal microalbuminuria ≥ 20 μg/minute, observed in 5.7% and 6.0% *vs* 10.0% of cases, respectively (p = 0.01 for the 2 comparisons). Verapamil SR 240 mg daily prescribed alone had a similar effect to that of placebo.

■ In the **ADVANCE** study conducted in 11,140 patients with type 2 diabetes, 68% of whom had already been treated for HT and 32% were normotensive, with a mean follow-up of 4.3 years, systematic addition of a fixed combination of perindopril 4 mg-indapamide 1.25 mg vs placebo to previous treatment decreased SBP and DBP by an average of 5.6 and 2.2 mmHg, respectively, decreased the relative risk of a major macrovascular or microvascular event (cardiovascular mortality, nonfatal stroke, nonfatal myocardial infarction, onset or deterioration of diabetic renal or ocular complications) by 9% (p = 0.04) and decreased cardiovascular mortality by 18% (p = 0.03) and all-cause mortality by 14% (p = 0.03). After 5 years, this treatment would prevent one death for every 79 patients treated.

■ In the **STAR** study conducted in 240 hypertensive patients with a mean age of 51.3 years and presenting a metabolic syndrome (fasting blood glucose between 1 and 1.25 g/L (5.5 and 6.9 mmol/L) and one of the following criteria: HDL-C < 0.40 g/L, i.e. 1.03 mmol/L in males and < 0.50 g/L, i.e. 1.29 mmol/L in females; triglycerides > 1.50 g/L, i.e. 1.71 mmol/L; waist > 102 cm in males and 89 cm in females), with a follow-up of 52 weeks, the fixed combination of trandolapril 2 mg daily + verapamil 180 mg daily vs the combination of losartan 50 mg daily + hydrochlorothiazide 12.5 mg daily, ensured significantly better control of blood glucose parameters: smaller elevation (p < 0.001) of blood glucose during the oral glucose load test (primary endpoint); lower frequency of HbA1c > 7% (2.6% vs 9.6%; p = 0.05); lower incidence of de novo diabetes (11.0% vs 26.6%; p = 0.002), lower plasma insulin (p = 0.025).

■ In high risk patients, the combination of an ACE inhibitor and an ARB (ramipril-telmisartan) does not improve the efficacy of the ACE inhibitor as to the prevention of major cardiovascular events when left ventricular dysfunction and/or heart failure are not present.

■ This was demonstrated by the **ONTARGET** study (see p. 25) which included 36% of diabetics.

■ Moreover, this combination increases the risk of hypotensive symptoms, syncope and renal dysfunction.

■ The combination of losartan and aliskiren, an orally active direct renin inhibitor, improves the renal prognosis of hypertensive patients with type 2 diabetes and nephropathy.

■ This was demonstrated by the **AVOID** study conducted in 599 patients of this type; with a follow-up of 6 months, *vs* placebo, the addition of aliskiren (150 mg daily for 3 months, then 300 mg daily) to optimal antihypertensive therapy including losartan 100 mg daily tended to decrease BP by 2/1 mmHg ($p = 0.08$; NS) and significantly reduced the mean urinary albumin/creatinine ratio by 20% ($p < 0.001$).

■ Although ACE inhibitors and ARBs have a similar renal protective effect on diabetic nephropathy, ACE inhibitors may be the only class to prevent early mortality.

■ This was the conclusion reached by the meta-analysis by **Strippoli** (see p. 62).

◆ *In primary and secondary prevention, management of all cardiovascular risk factors is essential and addition of a statin to standard therapy is recommended regardless of the baseline total cholesterol, as it significantly decreases the incidence of major cardiovascular events (see p. 70-71).*

Diabetes and dyslipidemia

■ Diabetes and dyslipidemia are frequently associated.

■ The characteristic lipid abnormalities of type 2 diabetes are: elevated triglycerides and free fatty acids, decreased HDL-C and little or no increase of total cholesterol and LDL-C.

■ The combination of diabetes and dyslipidemia significantly increases the cardiovascular risk.

Primary prevention

■ A 1 mmol/L (0.39 g/L) reduction of LDL-C is accompanied by a 23% reduction of the risk of myocardial infarction or coronary mortality, a 17% reduction of the risk of fatal or nonfatal stroke and a 12% reduction of all-cause mortality (p < 0.0001 for each risk).

■ This was demonstrated by the meta-analysis by **Baigent** based on 14 randomized trials comprising 90,056 patients treated with statins with a follow-up of 5 years.

Statins

■ In patients with type 2 diabetes and no history of coronary heart disease, addition of a statin to antidiabetic therapy significantly decreases the incidence of major cardiovascular events regardless of baseline total cholesterol, LDL-C and triglycerides (high or normal).

■ This was demonstrated by the study of 5,963 diabetic patients and 14,573 nondiabetic patients included in the **HPS** study; with a follow-up of 5.0 years, simvastatin 40 mg daily prescribed to both groups *vs* placebo very significantly reduced the risk of a first major coronary event by about 25% and the risk of a first major vascular event by 22% (p < 0.0001) in diabetic patients compared to nondiabetic patients. In 2,426 diabetic patients with normal or even low baseline total cholesterol (< 1.16 g/L [3.0 mmol/L]), simvastatin decreased the risk of vascular events by 27% (p = 0.0007). According to this study, simvastatin should therefore be systematically prescribed to all diabetic patients.

■ This was recently confirmed by the **CARDS** study conducted on a population of diabetic patients with normal baseline LDL-C (≤ 1.16 g/L), but who presented another cardiovascular risk factor (HT, smoking, retinopathy, microalbuminuria or macroalbuminuria); with a mean follow-up of 3.9 years, atorvastatin 10 mg daily *vs* placebo decreased the risk of a first major cardiovascular event (coronary mortality, nonfatal myocardial infarction, resuscitated cardiac arrest, hospitalization for unstable angina, myocardial revascularization, stroke) by 37%

(p = 0.001) and tended to decrease total mortality by 27% (p = 0.059; NS).

■ Similar findings were observed in the group of diabetic patients included in the **ASCOT-LLA** study, the lipid-lowering treatment arm of the double-blind **ASCOT** study conducted with a 2 x 2 factorial plan in 19,342 hypertensive patients. With a mean follow-up of 3.3 years, the addition of atorvastatin 10 mg daily *vs* placebo to antihypertensive therapy very significantly reduced the risk of the composite endpoint comprising nonfatal myocardial infarction and fatal coronary event by 36% (p = 0.0005) by the first year when total cholesterol was ≥ 2.51 g/L (6.5 mmol/L).

◆ *The target LDL-C in primary prevention is < 1 g/L (2.6 mmol/L) in patients with diabetes and dyslipidemia associated with another cardiovascular risk factor and/or microalbuminuria or more severe renal disease.*

Secondary prevention

Statins

■ In patients with type 2 diabetes and a history of cardio-vascular disease, addition of a statin to the treatment of diabetes significantly decreases the recurrence rate of cardiovascular events regardless of baseline total cholesterol, LDL-C and triglycerides (high or normal).

◆ *In the absence of a large-scale clinical trial of secondary prevention specifically conducted in patients with type 2 diabetes, this assertion is based exclusively on retrospective analysis of more than 5,000 diabetic patients included in 6 clinical trials:*

■ Retrospective analysis of data from 202 diabetic patients included in the **4S** study (4,444 patients), with a mean follow-up of 5.4 years, showed that simvastatin 20 to 40 mg daily *vs* placebo decreased the risk of coronary mortality and nonfatal myocardial infarction by 55% (*vs* 32% in the overall study population).

■ In the group of 586 diabetic patients included in the **CARE** study (4,159 patients), with a mean follow-up of 5 years, pravastatin 40 mg daily *vs* placebo decreased the risk of coronary mortality and nonfatal myocardial infarction by 25% (*vs* 23% in the overall study population).

■ In the group of 782 diabetic patients included in the **LIPID** study (9,014 patients), with a mean follow-up of 6.1 years, pravastatin 40 mg daily *vs* placebo decreased the risk of coronary mortality, nonfatal myocardial infarction and myocardial revascularization by 19% (*vs* 24% in the overall study population).

■ In the group of 5,963 diabetic patients included in the **HPS** study (20,536 patients), with a mean follow-up of 5 years, simvastatin 40 mg daily *vs* placebo decreased the risk of a major coronary event, stroke or myocardial revascularization by 18% (*vs* 24% in the overall study population).

■ In the group of 202 diabetic patients included in the **LIPS** study (1,677 patients), with a mean follow-up of 3.9 years, fluvastatin 80 mg daily *vs* placebo decreased the risk of coronary mortality, nonfatal myocardial infarction and myocardial revascularization by 47% (*vs* 22% in the overall study population).

■ In the group of 313 diabetic patients included in the **GREACE** study (1,600 patients), with a mean follow-up of 3 years, atorvastatin 10 to 80 mg daily *vs* placebo decreased the risk of coronary mortality, nonfatal myocardial infarction and myocardial revascularization, stroke and unstable angina by 58% (*vs* 51% in the overall study population).

■ Statins must therefore be systematically prescribed to all diabetic patients with a history of cardiovascular disease.

■ The target LDL-C in these patients is ≤ 0.70 g/L (1.8 mmol/L).

■ In diabetics with non-target LDL-C despite the maximum tolerated dose of statin, the addition of ezetimibe, a specific inhibitor of cholesterol absorption, can be helpful.

■ The combination of a statin and a fibrate or nicotinic acid can also be considered in some cases.

■ The absolute risk reduction provided by statins in patients with coronary heart disease and diabetes or simply impaired glucose tolerance is greater than that observed in normoglycemic patients with coronary heart disease.

■ Although statins decrease the relative risk of cardiovascular events to a similar degree in diabetic and nondiabetic patients with dyslipidemia and coronary heart disease, the absolute risk reduction is greater in diabetic patients and patients with impaired glucose tolerance as they are exposed to a higher rate of cardiovascular events than normoglycemic patients.

■ Retrospective analysis of the data of the **4S** study showed that, in patients with simply impaired glucose tolerance (fasting blood glucose between 1.10 g/L and 1.25 g/L [6.1 mmol/L and 6.93 mmol/L]), with a mean follow-up of 5.4 years, simvastatin 20-40 mg daily *vs* placebo decreased the relative risk of major coronary events by 38% (p = 0.003), coronary mortality by 55% (p = 0.007) and total mortality by 43% (p = 0.02).

Fibrates

■ The benefit effect of fibrates is more uncertain.

◆ *It appeared to be established by the **DAIS** study.*

■ In this primary and secondary prevention study (48% of patients had a history of coronary heart disease) conducted in 418 patients with type 2 diabetes and minor lipid abnormalities (total cholesterol/HDL-C ratio ≥ 4 with either LDL-C between 1.35 and 1.75 g/L [3.5 to 4.5 mmol/L], associated with triglycerides < 4.55 g/L [5.2 mmol/L], or triglycerides between 1.53 and 4.55 g/L [1.7 to 5.2 mmol/L] associated with LDL-C ≤ 1.75 g/L [4.51 mmol/L]), with a mean follow-up of 3 years, fenofibrate 200 mg daily *vs* placebo slowed progression of coronary atherosclerosis (40% reduction of progression of the minimum arterial lumen diameter of the qualifying stenosis). However, this study did not have sufficient power to assess the clinical consequences of these angiographic changes.

◆ *The results of the large-scale **FIELD** study are more mixed.*

■ In this study conducted in 9,795 patients with type 2 diabetes aged 50 to 75 years with (2,131 patients) or without (7,664 patients) a history of cardiovascular disease, with total cholesterol < 2.5 g/L (6.5 mmol/L), triglycerides < 4.35 g/L (5.0 mmol/L), a total cholesterol/HDL-C ratio ≥ 4.0, and not initially treated with statins, with a mean follow-up of 5.0 years, addition of fenofibrate 200 mg daily *vs* placebo to the treatment of diabetes tended to decrease the relative risk of the main composite endpoint comprising coronary mortality and nonfatal myocardial infarction by 11% (p = 0.16; NS), which corresponds to a significant 24% reduction (p = 0.010) of the nonfatal infarction rate, and tended to increase the fatal infarction rate by 19% (p = 0.22; NS). Fenofibrate also decreased the overall rate of cardiovascular events by 11% (p = 0.035) and especially the myocardial revascularization rate by 21% (p = 0.003) without affecting total mortality; it also slowed progression of albuminuria (p = 0.002) and the number of cases of retinopathy requiring laser therapy. This result was acquired at the price of a slight but significant increase of the risk of pancreatitis (0.8% *vs* 0.5%; p = 0.031) and pulmonary embolism (1.1% *vs* 0.7%; p = 0.022).

◆ *Consequently, the beneficial effect of fibrates in diabetic patients is much less clearly demonstrated than that of statins.*

Diabetes and coronary heart disease

■ Diabetes multiplies the risk of coronary heart disease by a factor of 2 to 4.

■ In the meta-analysis by **Lee**, based on 7 prospective studies comprising about 60,000 subjects aged 40 to 70 years, with no signs of coronary heart disease, with a follow-up of 4.5 to 20 years, the relative risk of coronary mortality was multiplied by 1.85 in male diabetics and by 2.37 in female diabetics compared to nondiabetic subjects.

■ Diabetics currently represent about 20% of all patients with coronary heart disease.

■ In the population of coronary patients included in the **EUROASPIRE II** study, 29% had known diabetes and 23% presented glucose intolerance.

■ Consequently, even in the absence of known diabetes, all patients with cardiovascular disease should be systematically evaluated by an oral glucose load test.

■ Coronary heart disease presents specific features in diabetics.

■ It is characterized by its latency (high frequency of silent myocardial ischemia), the extent and dissemination of anatomical lesions and by its rapid clinical course.

■ Diabetic patients have a higher risk of myocardial infarction than nondiabetic patients with a history of myocardial infarction.

■ In the study by **Haffner**, with a follow-up of 7 years, the incidence of myocardial infarction in nondiabetic subjects was 18.8% or 3.5%, respectively, according to whether or not they had a history of myocardial infarction; these percentages were much higher in diabetic patients: 45.0% and 20.2%, respectively (p < 0.001).

■ In acute myocardial infarction, blood glucose abnormalities must no longer be considered to be purely related to stress, as they are still present at the 3rd month in more than one half of cases.

■ These abnormalities therefore cannot all be attributed, as was thought for many years, to inhibition of insulin secretion due to excessive catecholamine secretion secondary to the initial acute stress.

■ Strict control of diabetes during the acute phase of myocardial infarction improves the medium-term and long-term prognosis.

■ This was demonstrated by the **DIGAMI 1** study conducted in 620 diabetic patients included during the first hours of myocardial infarction and treated by glucose and insulin infusion to maintain blood glucose between 1.26 and 1.98 g/L (7-11 mmol/L); in the medium term, with a mean follow-up of 3.4 years, continuation of insulin injections several times a day for at least 3 months significantly reduced mortality by 29% (p = 0.027).

■ The **DIGAMI 2** study conducted in 1,253 patients with type 2 diabetes, with a mean age of 68 years, did not confirm the results of the **DIGAMI 1** study: with a mean follow-up of 1.94 years initial intensive insulin therapy did not appear to be superior to oral antidiabetics and no difference was observed between treatment groups in terms of mortality and cardiovascular morbidity. These negative results can be explained by the improved management of the other cardiovascular risk factors in **DIGAMI 2**. However, this study recalled that blood glucose is an independent and powerful predictive factor of long-term post-infarction mortality, which is increased by 20% for a 0.54 g/L (3 mmol/L) elevation of blood glucose.

■ Type 2 diabetes worsens the short-term (hospital phase), medium-term and long-term prognosis of acute coronary syndromes, the treatment of which is based on the same principles as for nondiabetic patients.

Prevention of diabetes

■ Prevention of type 2 diabetes is now possible.

■ This prevention is based on a radical modification of the lifestyle of subjects at high risk of developing diabetes, with appropriate advice and, if necessary, pharmacological therapy. This strategy can reduce the risk of developing diabetes or can delay its onset.

■ Weight reduction associated with regular physical exercise decreases the risk of developing type 2 diabetes by 50%.

■ In the Chinese **Pan** study conducted in 110,600 male and female subjects with glucose intolerance, dietary measures associated with regular exercise, with a follow-up of 6 years, decreased the risk of developing type 2 diabetes by 42% (p < 0.005).

■ In the **Finnish diabetes prevention** study conducted in 522 subjects at high-risk of developing type 2 diabetes because of a body mass index ≥ 25 kg/m^2 and glucose intolerance, rigorous management (dietary advice associated with regular exercise) *vs* simple advice, with a follow-up of 4 years, decreased the relative risk of developing type 2 diabetes by 58% (10% *vs* 22%). Additional follow-up of the study for 3 years after stopping all intervention showed persistence of the acquired benefit.

■ Most importantly, this was very authoritatively demonstrated by the **DPP** study conducted in 3,234 patients with a mean age of 51 years, at high risk of developing type 2 diabetes because of glucose intolerance (blood glucose: 1.10-1.25 g/L [6.10-6.93 mmol/L]) and obesity (mean body mass index: 34 kg/m^2) possibly associated with a family history. With a follow-up of 3 years, dietary measures (7% weight loss, walking for 150 minutes/week) decreased the risk of diabetes by 58% (14% of patients in this group *vs* about 29% of patients in the control group).

■ The combination of drug therapy and a lifestyle modification program can prevent or delay the onset of type 2 diabetes in subjects with a disorder of blood glucose regulation at baseline.

■ Metformin, acarbose and rosiglitazone have demonstrated their efficacy in this indication. The same applies to orlistat.

■ This was demonstrated by the **STOP-NIDDM** study conducted in 1,429 patients with simple glucose intolerance. With a mean follow-up of 3.3 years, regular treatment with acarbose (target dosage: 100 mg x 3 daily) *vs* placebo significantly decreased the relative risk of diabetes by 25% (p = 0.0015) and increased the percentage of patients in whom glucose returned to normal (p < 0.0001).

■ In the **DREAM** study, rosiglitazone 15 mg daily decreased the risk of diabetes by 60%.

■ In the **XENDOS** study, orlistat reduced this risk by 37%.

■ In patients with hypertension, it has now been demonstrated that antihypertensive therapy by most ACE inhibitors or ARBs decreases the risk of diabetes by slightly more than 20% (*J Am Coll Cardiol* 2005; *46*: 821-826).

Metabolic syndrome
(European Recommendations, *Eur Heart J* 2003;24:1601-1610)

It is associated with a high cardiovascular risk. The diagnosis is based on the presence of at least 3 of the following 5 criteria, including hypertension:

1) waist > 102 cm in men and > 88 cm in women;

2) serum triglycerides $\geq$ 1.5 g/L (1.7 mmol/L);

3) serum HDL-C < 0.40 g/L (< 1 mmol/L) in men
   and < 0.50 g/L (< 1.3 mmol/L) in women;

4) blood pressure $\geq$ 130-85 mmHg;

5) blood glucose $\geq$ 1.10 g/L (6.1 mmol/L).

Management of the metabolic syndrome is essentially based on lifestyle and dietary measures (weight loss, regular physical exercise), possibly associated with drug treatment of hypertension, dyslipidemia or diabetes.

CHAPTER 4

Stable angina

Antianginal drugs

■ In monotherapy, the various therapeutic categories have demonstrated an equivalent efficacy on the frequency of angina and improvement of exercise tolerance.

■ This was the conclusion reached by many small studies conducted with nitrates, beta-blockers, calcium channel blockers, potassium channel activator (nicorandil) and trimetazidine which partially inhibits cellular fatty acid oxidation and which is the only antianginal drug with no hemodynamic action.

■ Recently, ivabradine (5 mg bid up titrated to 7.5 mg bid), the first selective If current inhibitor, which reduces heart rate and was found to possess superior anti-ischemic efficacy compared to placebo, was shown to be as effective as atenolol 50-100 mg daily in the **INITIATIVE** study conducted in 939 patients with stable angina.

■ Beta-blockers are usually prescribed as first-line therapy, but their beneficial effect on mortality has not been formally demonstrated.

■ This recommendation is based on extrapolation of the positive effect of beta-blockers demonstrated in post-myocardial infarction.

■ In fact, no mortality study has evaluated antianginal monotherapy *vs* placebo.

■ Antianginal combination therapy is usually reserved to failures of monotherapy.

■ In the **TRIMPOL II** study, the combination of trimetazidine 20 mg x 3 daily and metoprolol 5mg x 2 daily was more effective on exercise tolerance than metoprolol 50 mg x 2 daily alone.

◆ *According to ESC Guidelines 2006, metabolically acting agents protect from ischaemia by increasing glucose metabolism relative to that of fatty acids. Both trimetazidine and ranolazine, have been shown to have anti-anginal efficacy. They may be used in combination therapy with haemodynamically acting agents, as their primary effect is not through reduction in heart rate or blood pressure. Trimetazidine has been available for several years, but not in all countries. Wether these drugs influence the prognosis of patients with stable angina has not been determined.*

■ In the **IONA** study, the first large-scale morbidity and mortality study conducted in 5,126 patients with stable coronary heart disease, with a mean follow-up of 1.6 year, nicorandil prescribed in addition to another antianginal drug (beta-blocker or calcium channel blocker), decreased the risk of coronary mortality, myocardial infarction or emergency hospitalization for chest pain by 17% (p = 0.014), the risk of an acute coronary event by 21% (p = 0.028) and the risk of coronary mortality or myocardial infarction by 21% (NS).

■ In a second large-scale study, **ACTION**, nifedipine SR was compared to placebo in 7,665 patients with stable angina treated by beta-blockers or nitrates. In this study, with a mean follow-up of 4.9 years, nifedipine SR did not modify the major cardiovascular event-free survival but decreased the rate of coronary angiography and revascularization.

■ In the **CAMELOT** study conducted in 1,991 non-hypertensive patients with stable coronary heart disease without left ventricular dysfunction (LV ejection fraction > 40%), 3/4 of whom were treated by beta-blockers, amlodipine 10 mg daily significantly decreased (p = 0.003) the combined incidence of cardiovascular events *vs* placebo, while enalapril had a lesser and non-significant effect. The comparison between amlodipine and enalapril did not reveal any significant difference on the primary endpoint or on the other endpoints, apart from a reduction of hospitalizations for angina with amlodipine. However, a tendency in favor of amlodipine on revascularization and stroke rates, and a tendency in favor of enalapril on myocardial infarction and cardiovascular mortality were observed. Amlodipine also tended to decrease progression of atherosclerosis assessed by intracoronary ultrasound.

■ In the **ASSOCIATE** study, that was conducted in 889 patients already receiving beta-blockers, but still ischemic, ivabradine (5 mg bid up titrated to 7.5 mg bid after 2 months) was added on top of the optimal treatment. The addition to the beta-blocker of ivabradine 7.5 mg bid vs placebo for 4 months was well tolerated (only 1.1% of patient withdrew due to sinus bradycardia in the ivabradine group vs none with placebo) and led to a significant improvement in all parameters of exercise tolerance test at trough of drug activity compared to the beta-blocker alone.

■ In the recent **BEAUTIFUL** study that was conducted in 10,917 stable coronary patients with associated left ventricular dysfunction, already receiving current optimal preventive therapy, it was shown that patients who have a resting heart rate ≥ 70 beats per minute have a significantly higher risk of all major cardiovascular events. In these high risk patients (HR $\geq$ 70 bpm), the use of ivabradine (5 mg up to the target dose of 7.5 mg twice a day) (see p. 79) led to a significant reduction in risk of myocardial infarction by 36% ($p = 0.001$) and the need for coronary revascularization by 30% ($p = 0.016$), making ivabradine the only antianginal drug shown to reduce myocardial infarction in these patients.

Prophylaxis of acute ischemic events

■ This prophylaxis is based on the use of three drug classes, which should be an integral part of the prescription for all patients with coronary heart disease.

■ Aspirin decreases cardiovascular morbidity and mortality.

■ This was demonstrated by the **SAPAT** study and the **ATT** meta-analysis based on 7 trials comprising 2,920 patients. With a follow-up of 27 months, aspirin 75-150 mg daily significantly decreased the risk of cardiovascular mortality, myocardial infarction and stroke by 33%.

■ Statins decrease cardiovascular morbidity and mortality.

■ Although no studies have been specifically devoted to stable angina, secondary prevention with statins is known to decrease cardiovascular morbidity and mortality and total mortality (see p. 126).

■ A statin should be prescribed systematically, regardless of baseline cholesterol, in order to maintain LDL-C below 1 g/L.

■ Several studies, for example the **ALLIANCE**, **TNT** and **IDEAL** studies, appear to demonstrate the value of lowering LDL-C as much as possible (to 0.80 g/L or even lower) by using high doses of statins in high-risk patients (see p. 127).

■ ACE inhibitors decrease morbidity and mortality in patients with coronary heart disease, even in the absence of left ventricular dysfunction (see p. 128).

■ This beneficial effect, observed even in the absence of left ventricular dysfunction, has already been reported in post-myocardial infarction (**HOPE** study; see p. 36); it was confirmed by the **EUROPA** study (see p. 36).

■ This beneficial effect on cardiovascular risk was not observed in the **PEACE** study conducted in 8,290 patients with coronary heart disease, with intact left ventricular function (mean LVEF: 58%) receiving optimal therapy, as, with a mean follow-up of 4.8 years, the addition of trandolapril 4 mg daily *vs* placebo did not modify the risk of cardiovascular mortality, myocardial infarction and myocardial revascularization procedure (21.9% *vs* 22.5%; p = 0.43). In contrast, trandolapril reduced the incidence of hospitalization or death for heart failure (-25%; p = 0.02) and decreased the risk of *de novo* diabetes (-17%; p = 0.01).

■ The meta-analysis by **Dagenais** based on the **HOPE, EUROPA** and **PEACE** studies comprising a total of 29,805 patients, and the meta-analysis by **Danchin** based on 7 studies comprising a total of 33,960 coronary patients followed for 4.4 years confirmed that the addition of an ACE inhibitor to conventional therapy significantly reduced cardiovascular mortality and the major cardiovascular event rate.

The prescription for patients with stable coronary heart disease

■ It is similar to that for post-myocardial infarction and constitutes so-called BASIC therapy (see p. 125).

Myocardial revascularization

■ Revascularization is justified in refractory angina and improves the prognosis in certain indications.

■ Old studies and the meta-analysis by **Yusuf** showed that bypass graft (essentially venous) improved the prognosis compared to drug treatment alone in patients with positive ECG stress test with criteria of severity, left coronary common trunk stenosis, multivessel disease including a lesion of the proximal left anterior descending artery or associated with left ventricular dysfunction.

■ Coronary angioplasty improves angina and exercise tolerance, but its value to prevent myocardial infarction and decrease mortality has not been demonstrated in patients with single-vessel or two-vessel disease with no lesion of the proximal left anterior descending artery and without left ventricular dysfunction.

■ This was the conclusion reached by the **ACME, MASS, RITA 2, AVERT** studies and the meta-analysis by **Bucher**.

■ In patients with multivessel disease, coronary angioplasty and surgery globally have the same effect on the risk of death or myocardial infarction, but coronary angioplasty is less effective to suppress angina and iterative revascularizations.

■ This was demonstrated by 6 old studies (**RITA, GABI, EAST, CABRI, BARI, ERACI**) and the meta-analysis by **Pocock**, and by two more recent studies, **ARTS** and **SOS**.

■ In the recent **SYNTAX** study which randomized 1,800 patients with either left common trunk stenosis (isolated or associated with other lesions) or three-vessel disease, coronary artery bypass graft surgery appeared to be superior to angioplasty using Express Taxus active stents (an average of 4.6 stents per patient) in terms of the one-year incidence of the following events: death, stroke, myocardial infarction or revascularization (12.1% vs 17.8%; p = 0.0015). This difference was essentially due to a lower revascularization rate after coronary artery bypass graft (5.9% vs 13.7%; p < 0.001).

■ In diabetic patients with multivessel disease, surgery improves the prognosis compared to coronary angioplasty.

■ This was suggested by the **BARI** study and the meta-analysis by **Hoffman**.

■ However, in the recent **CARDIA** study which included 510 diabetic patients with multivessel disease, angioplasty (with active stents in 71% of patients) was equivalent to coronary artery bypass graft in terms of the one-year incidence of death, myocardial infarction or stroke (11.6% vs 10.2%; p = 063) at the price of a significantly higher subsequent revascularization rate (9.9% vs 2.0%; p = 0.001).

■ An initial strategy based on angioplasty in patients with stable coronary heart disease receiving optimal drug therapy does not modify the risk of death or infarction or other major cardiovascular events.

■ This was demonstrated by the recent **COURAGE** study which randomized 2,287 patients with a significant coronary lesion and angina or documented myocardial ischemia. Medical therapy comprised a platelet aggregation inhibitor (95% of cases), a beta-blocker (86%), a statin (93%) and an ACE inhibitor (64%). With a median follow-up of 4.6 years, angioplasty vs medical therapy alone did not modify the combined incidence of death or nonfatal infarction (19.0% vs 18.5%; p = 0.62), nor this primary endpoint combined with stroke (20.0% *vs* 19.5%; p = 0.62) nor the risk of myocardial infarction (13.2% *vs* 12.3%; p = 0.33). However, angioplasty was more effective to reduce angina symptoms.

Angina pectoris: functional classification		
	Canadian Cardiovascular Society (CCS[1])	**New York Heart Association (NYHA[2])**
• **Class I**	• Angina on violent, rapidly performed or prolonged physical activity or in sportsmen	• No angina for ordinary physical activity
• **Class II**	• Angina on rapid walking or on sloping ground or on flat ground after a meal or during cold or windy weather or emotional stress or in the morning after waking	• Angina on mild exertion
	• Angina on climbing more than one flight of stairs at normal speed	
• **Class III**	• Angina while walking on flat ground for less than two blocks	• Angina for less than ordinary physical activity
	• Angina on climbing a flight of stairs at normal speed	
• **Class IV**	• Angina on walking several steps or during personal hygiene or at rest	• Angina on the slightest exertion or at rest

(1) L. Campeau (*Circulation* 1976;*54*:522).
(2) The Criteria Committee of the New York Heart Association (*Diseases of the Heart and Blood Vessels. Nomenclature and Criteria for Diagnosis*, 6th ed., Boston, Little, Brown and Co., 1964).

EDRF, NO and nitrates

• **Furchgott**, **Ignarro** and **Murrad** received the 1998 Nobel Prize for having demonstrated that acetylcholine-induced vascular relaxation required the presence of endothelial cells and was mediated by EDRF (Endothelium Derived Relaxing Factor), an extremely labile substance (half-life: 3 to 50 seconds) synthesized by the endothelium, and identified EDRF to be nitric oxide (NO) synthesized by the endothelium from endogenous L-arginine (in the absence of L-arginine,endothelial cells loose their capacity to release NO;administration of L-arginine corrects this situation).

• Under physiological conditions, vascular endothelium releases EDRF alias NO, which acts as an endogenous nitrate and induces vasodilatation.

• In contrast, in the presence of ischemic heart disease, accompanied by an anatomical or functional alteration of the endothelium, EDRF alias NO is no longer able to ensure its role, possibly because of its very rapid degradation related to the presence of excess oxygen-derived free radicals produced by the altered endothelium. Under these pathological conditions, nitroglycerin behaves as an exogenous NO donor on vascular smooth muscle fibers.

European guidelines on the treatment of stable angina pectoris
(Eur Heart J 2006;27:1341-1381)

- After initial risk evaluation, risk-factor correction by life-style modification should be implemented in addition to pharmacological intervention as necessary. Strict diabetic control and weight control along with smoking cessation strategies are strongly advised in all patients with coronary disease, and blood pressure control is extremely important. Successful risk-factor management may modify the initial risk assessment.

- In terms of specific pharmacological therapy, short-acting nitrates, when tolerated, may be used to provide acute symptomatic relief. In the absence of contraindications or intolerance, patients with stable angina pectoris should be treated with aspirin (75 mg/day) and statin therapy. A beta-blocker should be used first line or,alternatively, an If inhibitor, a calcium-channel blocker or a long-acting nitrate may be used to provide anti-anginal effects, with additional therapy as necessary. ACE-inhibition is indicated in patients with co-existing ventricular dysfunction, hypertension, or diabetes and should be strongly considered in patients with other high-risk features. Beta-blockers should be recommended in all post-MI patients and in patients with LV dysfunction, unless contraindicated. Metabolic agents such as trimetazidine may be used as add-on therapy, or as substitution therapy when conventional drugs are not tolerated.

- Anti-anginal drug treatment should be tailored to the needs of the individual patient and should be monitored individually. The dosing of one drug should be optimized before adding another one, and it is advisable to switch drug combinations before attempting a three drug regimen.

- If not undertaken for further prognostic evaluation, coronary arteriography should be undertaken when symptoms are no satisfactorily controlled by medical means, with a view to revascularization.

- PCI is an effective treatment for stable angina pectoris and is indicated for patients with angina not satisfactorily controlled by medical treatment when there are anatomically suitable lesions. Restenosis continues to be a problem, which has been diminished by advances in stenting technology. There is no evidence that PCI reduces the risk of death in patients with stable angina compared with medical or surgical therapy.

- CABG is highly effective in relieving the symptoms of stable angina and reduces the risk of death over long-term follow-up in particular subgroups of patients, such as those with LM stem stenosis, proximal LAD stenosis, and three-vessel disease, especially if LV function is impaired.

- There is evidence that some gaps remain between best practice and usual care in the management of stable angina. Specifically, many individuals with stable angina are not referred for functional testing to confirm the diagnosis and determine prognosis. Furthermore, there is worrying variability in rates of prescription of statins and aspirin. Because of the wide variations in the quality of care afforded to sufferers from angina, there is a strong case for auditing several components of the management of the condition. As is the practice in some countries, local, regional, or national registers of the outcome of PCI and surgery should be created and maintained.

CHAPTER 5

Acute coronary syndrome without persistent ST-segment elevation

Factual data

■ The essential mechanism, common to the various acute coronary syndromes (ACS), is rupture or fissure of an atheromatous plaque leading to the formation of coronary thrombosis.

  ■ Lesions likely to rupture generally induce moderate, insignificant stenoses, corresponding to immature plaques with a lipid-rich histological structure, composed of a soft atheromatous nucleus covered by a fine, fragile, fibrous shell, presenting signs of inflammation.

  ■ The consequence of plaque rupture is the formation of thrombus, usually a nonocclusive fibrin and platelet thrombus in ACS without persistent ST-segment elevation, to which are added vasospastic phenomena.

  ■ Sudden reduction of the epicardial arterial lumen is frequently associated with occlusion of distal arterioles by platelet emboli shed by the unstable plaque.

■ The new classification of ACS distinguishes myocardial infarction without persistent ST-segment elevation (formerly, non-Q wave myocardial infarction) in the presence of elevated troponin and unstable angina when there is no elevation of markers of myocardial necrosis.

■ ACS without persistent ST-segment elevation is about twice as frequent as acute myocardial infarction with ST elevation.

■ This was demonstrated by the **GRACE** prospective register, in which unstable angina represented 38% of cases, myocardial infarction without persistent ST-segment elevation represented 25% of cases and myocardial infarction with persistent ST-segment elevation represented 30% of cases (diagnosis of ACS not confirmed in the remaining 7% of cases).

■ ACS without persistent ST-segment elevation corresponds to several clinical presentations that do not have the same prognostic significance.

■ It may consist of spontaneous angina, accelerated exertional angina, *de novo* exertional angina or post-myocardial infarction angina.

■ After risk stratification, antithrombotic therapy and usually myocardial revascularization prevent progression to myocardial infarction with persistent ST-segment elevation or sudden death in more than 90% of patients.

Risk stratification

■ Risk stratification, performed within 24 hours after admission, guides the choice between an early invasive strategy and a conservative strategy.

■ The invasive strategy consists of performing coronary angiography during the first days of the acute episode, followed by revascularization (angioplasty or bypass graft) whenever anatomically possible. The conservative strategy consists of performing coronary angiography and revascularization only in the case of spontaneous recurrent ischemia despite well conducted treatment or demonstration of residual ischemia on a stress test performed at the end of hospitalization or after discharge.

■ Risk stratification is based on clinical, electrocardiographic, laboratory and echocardiographic parameters.

■ Parameters indicating a possible unfavorable outcome are:

– Clinical parameters: angina at rest, the repeated and recent nature of angina attacks, incomplete response to medical treatment, advanced age, accelerated heart rate, low blood pressure and heart failure.

– ECG parameters: ST-segment depression on admission, but also transient and silent episodes of ST-segment depression or elevation.

– Laboratory parameters: even minimal elevation of troponin confirmed on 2 assays at an interval of 6 hours.

– Echocardiographic parameters: presence of left ventricular systolic dysfunction.

■ Simple and reliable risk scores have been defined.

■ For example, the **TIMI** risk score attributes 1 point to each of the following 7 variables: age $\geq$ 65 years, presence of at least 3 risk factors for coronary heart disease, documented coronary artery stenosis, ST depression on baseline ECG, presence of at least 2 episodes of angina during the previous 24 hours, aspirin treatment during the previous 7 days and elevation of laboratory markers of myocardial necrosis.

■ This score, established on the basis of the **TIMI 11B** study, then validated by several large-scale studies, shows that the risk of death, reinfarction or severe recurrent ischemia at 14 days is 4.7% for a score of 0 or 1 point, 8.3% for 2 points, 13.2% for 3 points, 19.9% for 4 points, 26.2% for 5 points and 40.9% for 6 or 7 points.

Early invasive strategy *vs* conservative strategy

■ Progress in coronary angioplasty has demonstrated the superiority of the early invasive strategy in high- or intermediate-risk patients.

◆ *However, the first studies conducted before the age of stents and GP IIb/IIIa receptor inhibitors were not conclusive.*

■ The **TIMI IIIB** and **VANQWISH** studies indicated that a systematic invasive strategy had a neutral or even a negative impact.

◆ *Three large-scale studies have demonstrated the value of revascularization in high-risk patients.*

■ In the **FRISC II** study, which included 2,457 patients ≤ 75 years, the invasive strategy decreased the rate of death or myocardial infarction (9.4% *vs* 12.1%; p = 0.031), the incidence of angina (22% *vs* 39%; p < 0.001), readmissions (31% *vs* 49%; p < 0.001) and late revascularizations (5.6% *vs* 23.0%; p < 0.001) at the 6th month. The beneficial effect was even more marked at one year, with a significant reduction of mortality (2.2% *vs* 3.9%; p = 0.016) and myocardial infarction (8.6% *vs* 11.6%; p = 0.015). Despite a higher rate of severe bleeding (1.6% *vs* 0.7%), the invasive strategy did not increase the incidence of stroke and intracranial hemorrhage.

■ In the **TACTICS-TIMI 18** study, which included 2,220 patients with a mean age of 62 years, all treated with a GP IIb/IIIa receptor inhibitor, the invasive strategy, compared to the conservative strategy, significantly decreased the combined rate of death, myocardial infarction or readmission for ACS in 6 months (15.9% *vs* 19.4%; p = 0.025); this difference essentially concerned recurrent myocardial infarction (4.8% *vs* 6.9%; p = 0.029). The invasive strategy did not modify the incidence of either stroke or major bleeding.

■ In the **RITA 3** study conducted in 1,810 patients with a mean age of 62 years, the invasive strategy significantly decreased the rate of death, myocardial infarction or refractory angina at

4 months (9.6% *vs* 14.5%); this difference was mainly related to a 50% reduction of refractory angina.

◆ *That was confirmed by two recent meta-analyses.*

■ The meta-analysis by **Bavry** based on 5 studies comprising 6,766 patients, suggested that, in the age of stents and GP IIb/IIIa receptor inhibitors, the invasive strategy improved survival at 6 and 12 months.

■ The meta-analysis by **Mehta** based on 7 studies comprising 9,212 patients with a follow-up of 17 months showed that the invasive strategy was superior to the conservative strategy, by significantly reducing the rate of myocardial infarction ($p < 0.001$), severe angina ($p < 0.001$) and readmissions ($p < 0.001$).

◆ *However, the recent ICTUS study has raised a doubt.*

■ In this study conducted in 1,200 high-risk patients with a follow-up of one year, the invasive strategy did not modify the combined incidence of death, nonfatal myocardial infarction or readmissions for angina. Early introduction of the most modern treatments, especially clopidogrel and high-dose statins, could explain the more favorable than expected outcome in the conservative strategy group.

■ In practice, certain parameters indicate the need for an early invasive strategy.

■ For **American and European Societies**, these parameters are: ST-segment depression on admission; recurrent angina or dynamic ST-segment changes; early unstable angina after myocardial infarction; elevation of troponin; hemodynamic instability; malignant ventricular arrhythmia; diabetes; ECG unable to evaluate ST-segment changes; coronary angioplasty during the previous 6 months; history of coronary artery bypass graft; systolic ventricular dysfunction (LVEF < 40%).

■ The invasive strategy can be performed very rapidly.

■ In the **ISAR-COOL** study conducted in 410 high-risk patients (ST-segment depression or elevated troponin) already treated with four-agent antithrombotic therapy (aspirin, clopidogrel, tirofiban and heparin), a very early invasive strategy (mean: 2.4 hours) compared to a deferred procedure (mean: 86 hours) significantly decreased the 30-day death or myocardial infarction rate (5.9% *vs* 11.6%; p = 0.04).

■ A conservative strategy can be proposed in low-risk patients (TIMI score 0-2, see p. 102), who represent about 1/4 of all cases of ACS without persistent ST-segment elevation.

■ This was demonstrated by the **FRISC II** and **TACTICS-TIMI 18** studies, in which the invasive strategy did not modify the incidence of death or myocardial infarction. However, it was more effective on prevention of recurrent angina.

Antithrombotic therapy

■ Whether an invasive or a conservative strategy is decided, antithrombotic therapy, started as soon as possible, has an essential place in the treatment of ACS without persistent ST-segment elevation.

Aspirin

■ Aspirin decreases progression to myocardial infarction and cardiac mortality by one half.

■ This was the conclusion reached by 4 placebo-controlled studies: the **Veterans Administration** study which included 1,266 patients, the **Canadian Multicenter Trial** conducted in 555 patients, the study by **Théroux** conducted in 479 patients and the **RISC** study conducted in 796 patients.

■ Meta-analysis of these 4 studies (*J Am Coll Cardiol* 2000; *36*: 970-1062) showed that aspirin very significantly decreased the risk of death or myocardial infarction at 5 days to 2 years depending on the study (6.4% *vs* 12.5%; p = 0.0005).

■ Low-dose aspirin (75-160 mg daily) is as effective as higher dosages, which increase the incidence of gastrointestinal adverse effects.

■ In the **RISC** study, aspirin 75 mg daily *vs* placebo decreased the combined risk of death and myocardial infarction by 57% at the 5th day, 69% at the 30th day, 64% at the 3rd month and 48% at one year. These results are at least equivalent to those obtained with higher dosages (325 to 1300 mg daily) in other studies.

■ However, to obtain a rapid effect of aspirin, an initial loading dose of 250-500 mg is recommended.

Clopidogrel

■ In the thienopyridine family, clopidogrel has supplanted ticlopidine because of its better hematologic safety and a comparable efficacy.

■ Clopidrogel must be prescribed in addition to aspirin.

■ Clopidogrel, started on the first day at a loading dose (300 mg) and continued for 9 months (75 mg daily), decreases major ischemic complications, independently of the severity of the ACS and whether or not coronary angioplasty is performed.

■ This was the conclusion of the **CURE** study conducted in 12,562 patients treated with aspirin, in whom clopidogrel *vs* placebo significantly decreased the combined incidence of cardiovascular mortality, nonfatal myocardial infarction or stroke by 20% for a mean follow-up of 9 months (9.3% *vs* 11.4%; p < 0.001); the most marked effect was observed for prevention of myocardial infarction.

■ The beneficial effect of clopidogrel was observed by the very first hours of treatment and the relative reduction of the vascular risk was comparable for the first 30 days and between the 30th day and the end of the study, indicating the value of continuing this treatment for several months.

■ In the context of an invasive strategy, clopidogrel, started several days before coronary angioplasty, associated with aspirin and continued for 9 months, decreases major cardiovascular events compared to treatment for only 4 weeks started on the day of the procedure.

■ This was demonstrated by the **PCI-CURE** study based on 2,658 patients of the **CURE** study dilated a median of 10 days after initial randomization between clopidogrel and placebo. At one month, clopidogrel administered rapidly with an initial loading dose significantly reduced the rate of cardiovascular mortality or myocardial infarction (2.9% *vs* 4.4%; p = 0.04) and continuation of clopidogrel beyond the first month after angioplasty decreased the incidence of the same events with a mean follow-up of 8 months (6.0% *vs* 8.0%; p = 0.047).

■ It is recommended to administer the loading dose of clopidogrel at least 6 hours before coronary angioplasty.

■ This was the conclusion reached by the **CREDO** study, which was not specifically devoted to ACS and which compared, in 2,116 patients, the standard clopidogrel protocol (75 mg daily, started immediately after coronary angioplasty and continued for 28 days) with pretreatment based on a loading dose of 300 mg of clopidogrel administered 3 to 24 hours before the procedure, and which was then continued at the dose of 75 mg daily for one year.

■ On the 28th day, pretreatment by clopidogrel significantly decreased the combined risk of death, myocardial infarction or another urgent revascularization by 38.6%, exclusively when the loading dose was administered at least 6 hours before coronary angioplasty.

■ Prolonged treatment compared to treatment for 28 days also decreased the combined risk of death, myocardial infarction or stroke by 26.9% (p = 0.02) at one year.

■ A loading dose of 600 mg of clopidogrel should be used in patients about to undergo an invasive procedure.

■ It is recommended to coprescribe clopidogrel with aspirin at a dose ≤ 100 mg daily and to stop clopidogrel at least 5 days before elective coronary surgery due to the increased bleeding risk.

■ Although major bleeding was more frequent with clopidogrel than with placebo (3.7% *vs* 2.7%; p = 0.001) in the **CURE** study, there was no significant increase of potentially fatal bleeding or intracranial hemorrhage and a dose of aspirin ≤ 100 mg daily did not increase the bleeding risk.

■ In the same study, hemorrhagic complications during coronary artery bypass graft were more frequent (9.6 vs 6.3% with placebo; p = 0.06), only when clopidogrel was stopped less than 5 days before surgery.

Prasugrel

■ Prasugrel, a new thienopyridine, is more effective than clopidogrel to prevent ischemic events related to angioplasty but it increases the major bleeding risk.

■ This was the conclusion of the **TRITON-TIMI 38** study which included 13,608 patients with moderate-or high-risk ACS and scheduled for angioplasty and stenting (active stent in 50% of cases). Prasugrel (10 mg daily after a loading dose of 60 mg) vs clopidogrel (75 mg daily after a loading dose of 300 mg), administered for 6 to 15 months, decreased the combined incidence of cardiovascular mortality, myocardial infarction or stroke by 19% (9.9% vs 12.1%; p < 0.001) and the incidence of myocardial infarction (7.4% vs 9.7%; p < 0.001) and stent thrombosis (1.1% vs 2.4%; p < 0.001), but at the price of excess major bleeding (2.4% vs 1.8%; p = 0.03), including fatal bleeds (0.4% vs 0.1%; p = 0.002).

Anticoagulants

■ Anticoagulation is recommended in all patients in combination with platelet aggregation inhibitor therapy.

■ Unfractionated heparin (UFH) is effective, especially in combination with aspirin.

■ This was the conclusion of the meta-analysis by **Oler** based on 6 trials comprising 1,356 patients. Compared to aspirin used alone, the heparin-aspirin combination decreased the risk of myocardial infarction or death during the randomization period by 33%, but with an increased bleeding risk.

■ Discontinuation of heparin therapy has been considered to frequently induce recurrence of the clinical syndrome, but this rebound phenomenon is only really observed in the absence of concomitant aspirin therapy.

■ **LMWH can replace UFH and enoxaparin is usually preferred.**

◆ *This was demonstrated by the **FRISC**, **FRIC**, **FRAXIS**, **ESSENCE** and **TIMI 11B** studies.*

■ In the **FRISC** study, which included 1,506 patients receiving aspirin 75 mg daily, dalteparin was shown to be superior to placebo by significantly decreasing the rate of myocardial infarction or death during the first 6 days (1.8% vs 4.8%; p = 0.001); the absolute benefit was maintained at the 40th day.

■ The **FRIC** study conducted in 1,482 patients and the **FRAXIS** study which included 3,468 patients showed that dalteparin and nadroparin gave equivalent results to those of UFH.

■ Only enoxaparin was demonstrated to be superior to UFH in the **ESSENCE** study and in the **TIMI 11B** study. The meta-analysis by **Antman** based on these 2 trials, comprising a total of 7,081 patients, showed that enoxaparin vs UFH significantly decreased the incidence of death or myocardial infarction at the 8th day (4.1% vs 5.3%; p = 0.02), 14th day (5.2% vs 6.5%; p = 0.02) and 43rd day (7.1% vs 8.6%; p = 0.02), without increasing the major bleeding risk.

■ **Continuation of LMWH therapy after discharge from hospital does not appear to provide any additional benefit.**

■ This was demonstrated by the **TIMI 11B** and **FRISC II** studies and by the meta-analysis by **Eikelboom** based on 5 trials comprising 12,099 patients, as long-term treatment significantly increased the major bleeding risk.

■ **Fondaparinux was shown to be equivalent to enoxaparin while reducing the bleeding risk by 50%.**

■ This was the conclusion of the **OASIS 5** study which included 20,078 patients. This study led to the recommendation of fondaparinux rather than enoxaparin in non-urgent situations (when the decision between a conservative or invasive strategy has not been made) in patients with a moderate or high bleeding risk. Enoxaparin is recommended for patients with a low bleeding risk.

■ Bivalirudin was shown to be superior to UFH and LMWH associated with GP IIb/IIIa receptor inhibitors in the context of angioplasty.

■ This was the conclusion of the **ACUITY** study which included 13,819 patients. In the emergency invasive setting, it is recommended to use either UFH, enoxaparin, or bivalirudin.

GP IIb/IIIa receptor inhibitors

■ A GP IIb/IIIa receptor inhibitor can be coprescribed with aspirin and heparin whenever angioplasty is considered.

■ This was the conclusion of 6 large-scale studies and the meta-analyses by **Roffi** and **Boersma**.

■ These studies evaluated eptifibatide in 10,948 patients (**PURSUIT** study), tirofiban in 5,147 patients (**PRISM** and **PRISM PLUS** studies), abciximab in 7,800 patients (**GUSTO IV-ACS** study) and lamifiban in 7,507 patients (**PARAGON A and B** studies).

■ The meta-analysis by **Roffi** demonstrated that:

– Globally, GP IIb/IIIa receptor inhibitors have a significant but moderate favorable effect on prevention of ischemic events with 8 deaths or infarctions avoided per 1,000 patients treated.

– A more marked benefit was observed when coronary angioplasty was performed during hospitalization (20 deaths or infarctions avoided per 1,000 patients treated), especially when the GP IIb/IIIa receptor inhibitor infusion was started before coronary angioplasty (31 events avoided per 1,000 patients treated).

– The benefit was limited and not significant in the absence of angioplasty, with 4 events avoided per 1,000 patients treated.

■ The benefit of GP IIb/IIIa receptor inhibitors depends on the risk level established on initial stratification and is particularly marked in diabetic patients.

■ In the meta-analysis by **Boersma**, the GP IIb/IIIa receptor inhibitor only decreased the 30-day incidence of death or infarction in the case of elevated troponin.

■ In the meta-analysis by **Roffi**, the benefit was particularly marked in diabetic patients, with a 26% reduction of mortality at one month, and a 70% reduction of mortality in combination with coronary angioplasty.

■ GP IIb/IIIa receptor inhibitors increase the bleeding risk, without modifying the incidence of intracranial hemorrhage.

■ This was demonstrated by the meta-analysis by **Boersma**, which reported an excess of major bleeding (2.4% vs 1.4%; p < 0.0001), but no increase of intracranial hemorrhage (0.09% vs 0.06%). This justifies compliance with the hemorrhagic contraindications, which are similar to those of IV thrombolysis in acute myocardial infarction.

■ Only tirofiban and eptifibatide can be used in the absence of coronary angioplasty.

■ The **GUSTO IV-ACS** study, which evaluated abciximab in 7,800 patients with no intention of revascularization during the first 48 hours, reported an early excess mortality and an increased bleeding risk with abciximab.

Anti-ischemic therapy

Nitrates

■ It is recommended to use an IV nitrate at a low starting dose, rapidly replaced by percutaneous or oral therapy.

■ In fact, no randomized placebo-controlled studies have been conducted with nitrates and related drugs.

Beta-blockers

■ Beta-blockers decrease the risk of progression to myocardial infarction.

■ This was the conclusion of the meta-analysis by **Yusuf** based on 7 trials comprising about 5,000 patients, in whom beta-blockers significantly decreased the incidence of infarction by 13% (29% *vs* 32%; p = 0.04), without modifying mortality.

■ In fact, no large-scale morbidity and mortality trial has studied the value of beta-blockers and the justification for their use is based on extrapolation of the beneficial effects observed in other clinical settings of ischemic heart disease.

◆ *In the absence of the usual contraindications, it is therefore recommended to systematically prescribe a beta-blocker as early as possible, reserving the IV route for high-risk patients with persistent pain.*

Calcium channel blockers

■ Calcium channel blockers globally have a neutral impact on prognosis.

■ This was demonstrated by the meta-analysis by **Held** based on 6 trials comprising 1,100 patients mostly treated with nifedipine.

■ Dihydropyridines must be avoided unless they are prescribed in combination with a beta-blocker.

■ This was the conclusion of the **HINT** study, in which short-acting nifedipine tended to increase the risk of early infarction compared to placebo.

■ However, no large-scale trial has evaluated third generation dihydropyridines in this indication.

■ Heart-rate-lowering calcium channel blockers can be used in the absence of left ventricular dysfunction, when beta-blockers are contraindicated.

■ This was demonstrated by several small studies, such as the **DRS** study, which evaluated diltiazem, and the **DAVIT II** study, which tested verapamil.

Coronary angioplasty *vs* coronary artery bypass graft

■ Classically, coronary artery bypass graft is superior to coronary angioplasty in certain indications, such as common trunk stenosis and threevessel disease, especially in the presence of left ventricular dysfunction or diabetes.

■ This was the conclusion of the meta-analysis by **Sim** based on 56 trials comprising 2,943 patients with multivessel disease, which demonstrated the equivalence between coronary artery bypass graft and balloon catheter coronary angioplasty in terms of intermediate-term mortality and infarction, although the repeat revascularization rate was much higher after coronary angioplasty.

■ In the **BARI** study, which included 1,829 patients with multivessel disease, 2/3 of whom presented unstable angina, coronary artery bypass graft improved the 7-year infarction-free survival (84.4% *vs* 80.9%; p = 0.04), but only in diabetic patients.

■ The superiority of surgery in patients with multivessel disease has been questioned with the progress in coronary angioplasty.

■ Recent studies, such as **ARTS** conducted in 1,205 patients, **ERACI II** conducted in 450 patients and **SOS** conducted in 988 patients, have reported contradictory results.

■ In the current state of knowledge, the 2 methods appear to be equivalent in terms of medium-term prognosis, and the higher cost of surgery is compensated by the cost of more numerous repeat revascularization procedures after angioplasty because of restenosis phenomena, especially in diabetics. New comparative studies are therefore necessary to evaluate coated stents, which considerably decrease restenosis phenomena.

Other drugs

Statins

■ Statins improve the coronary patient's prognosis, regardless of total cholesterol level.

■ This was largely demonstrated by the **4S, CARE, LIPID** and **HPS** studies (see p. 44-46).

■ Statins must be started in hospital to increase the long-term prescription and compliance rates.

■ A high dose of statin prescribed at the acute phase could reduce early ischemic complications and improve the long-term prognosis.

◆ *This was suggested by the* **MIRACL** *and* **PROVE-IT** *studies but the results of the* **A-to-Z** *study were less conclusive (see p. 46-47).*

■ In the arm of the **A-to-Z** study conducted in 4,497 patients hospitalized for acute coronary syndrome, with a follow-up of 2 years, simvastatin 40 mg daily for the first month then 80 mg daily only tended (p = 0.14; NS) to decrease the risk of the composite endpoint comprising death, myocardial infarction and recurrence of acute coronary syndrome or stroke *vs* placebo taken for 4 months then replaced by simvastatin 20 mg daily.

◆ *Meta-analysis of the* **PROVE-IT** *and* **A-to-Z** *studies recommended the use of high doses of statins.*

■ In the meta-analysis by **Murphy**, based on 8,658 patients, high-dose statins lowered LDL-C by an average of 0.64 g/L at the 8th month and induced a significant 23% reduction of total mortality compared to usual dosages (3.6% *vs* 4.9%; p = 0.015); this result appeared to be concordant in the various subgroups analyzed.

■ The increased incidence of adverse effects related to high doses of statin is compensated by their benefit on prognosis.

■ This was the conclusion of the meta-analysis by **Silva**, based on 27,548 patients with coronary heart disease included in 4 studies comparing a dose of 80 mg of atorvastatin or simvastatin to usual dosages. Although the risk of elevation of hepatic enzymes (> 3 times the upper limit of normal) was multiplied by 4.48 and the risk of elevation of CPK (> 10 times the upper limit of normal) was multiplied by 9.97, high-dose statins decreased cardiovascular mortality by 14% (p = 0.031), myocardial infarction by 16% (p < 0.001) and stroke by 18% (p = 0.004).

Angiotensin-converting enzyme (ACE) inhibitors

■ ACE inhibitors must be part of the discharge prescription, even in the absence of left ventricular systolic dysfunction.

Although no study has been specifically devoted to ACE inhibitors prescribed at the acute phase of ACS without persistent ST-segment elevation, the **HOPE** study (see p. 20) conducted with ramipril and the **EUROPA** study (see p. 36) conducted with perindopril, in patients without heart failure or left ventricular dysfunction, showed a preventive effect of the ACE inhibitor on the long-term incidence of a major cardiovascular event.

TIMI risk score in ACS without persistent ST-segment elevation
(*Circulation* 1999; *100*: 1593-1601)

● The score attributes 1 point to each of the following 7 variables:
  • age ≥ 65 years
  • at least 3 risk factors for coronary heart disease
  • already documented coronary stenosis > 50%
  • ST-segment depression on baseline ECG
  • at least 2 episodes of angina during the previous 24 hours
  • aspirin treatment during the previous 7 days
  • elevation of laboratory markers of myocardial necrosis

● Risk of death, (re)infarction or emergency revascularization for severe recurrent ischemia within 14 days
  • low: score 0 to 2
  • intermediate: score 3 to 4
  • high: score 5 to 7

CHAPTER 6

Myocardial infarction with persistent ST-segment elevation

Factual data

■ Nine factors can predict 90% of the risk of myocardial infarction.

■ This was demonstrated by the **INTERHEART** case-control study conducted in 52 countries and comparing 14,820 healthy subjects with 15,152 patients experiencing a first myocardial infarction. The 6 negative prognostic factors were: an abnormal apo B/apo A1 ratio, smoking, diabetes, hypertension, abdominal obesity and unfavorable psychosocial factors. The 3 protective factors were: daily consumption of fruit and vegetables, regular physical exercise and moderate alcohol consumption.

Early restoration of coronary perfusion

■ This is the best way to ensure a good prognosis.

■ It has been generally accepted since the studies by **Falk, Davies** and **Dewood** that occlusive coronary thrombosis is responsible for acute myocardial infarction in more than 90% of cases.

Early restoration of coronary perfusion, by means of IV thrombolysis or coronary angioplasty, is the best way to improve the prognosis, as it limits the extent of necrosis and consequently preserves left ventricular function.

Intravenous thrombolysis

■ IV thrombolysis decreases mortality in patients treated during the first 12 hours after myocardial infarction.

■ This was the conclusion of studies conducted with the first 3 fibrinolytics evaluated *vs* placebo, i.e. streptokinase in the **GISSI** and **ISIS 2** trials, alteplase in the **AIMS** study and anistreplase in the **AIMS** study.

■ The gain in terms of prognosis is greater when thrombolysis is initiated rapidly after onset of symptoms.

■ This was demonstrated by the meta-analysis by **Boersma**, in which the number of lives saved was 65,37 and 26 per 1,000 patients treated at the 1st, 2nd and 3rd hour of myocardial infarction, respectively. In the **GISSI** study, the maximum reduction of mortality was 50% in patients treated during the first hour of infarction, also called the "golden hour".

◆ *This emphasizes the importance of prehospital thrombolysis, initiated at the patient's home.*

■ The **EMIP** study, performed in 5,469 patients randomized during the first 6 hours of myocardial infarction, showed that prehospital thrombolysis compared to thrombolysis performed on arrival at hospital, gained 55 minutes and was accompanied by a significant reduction of cardiac mortality at the time of discharge (8.3% *vs* 9.8%). Similarly, the meta-analysis by **Morrison** based on 6 randomized studies including a total of 6,434 patients confirmed that prehospital thrombolysis gained about 1 hour and was accompanied by a significant 17% reduction of hospital mortality in relative values, compared to treatment started on arrival at hospital.

◆ *The time to initiation of thrombolysis can nevertheless be extended until the 12th hour.*

■ This was the conclusion of the **LATE** study, which included 5,711 patients with myocardial infarction evolving for 6 to 24 hours. IV thrombolysis by alteplase *vs* placebo decreased the mortality at the 35th day, but exclusively in patients treated between the 6th and 12th hour: 8.9% *vs* 12.0%, i.e. a relative reduction of 25% (p = 0.02).

■ The benefit of thrombolysis is significant regardless of age (at least before the age of 75), gender, blood pressure, heart rate, presence or absence of a history of myocardial infarction or diabetes.

■ This was the conclusion of the **FTT collaborative group** meta-analysis based on 9 studies comprising 58,600 patients.

■ The absolute benefit of thrombolysis is even greater in high-risk patients.

■ This was demonstrated by the **FTT collaborative group** meta-analysis.

■ Although the relative reduction of mortality, about 20%, was similar in the various patient subgroups analyzed, the absolute benefit expressed in number of lives saved was considerably higher in patients with a spontaneous high risk. The number of lives saved per 1,000 patients treated was 49 in the presence of bundle branch block, 37 in the case of anterior myocardial infarction (*vs* 8 in the case of inferior myocardial infarction), 27 in patients aged 65 to 74 years (*vs* 11 in patients younger than 55), 62 when SBP was < 100 mmHg, 33 when heart rate was ≥ 100 bpm (*vs* 13 when heart rate was < 80 bpm), and 37 in the presence of diabetes (*vs* 15 in the absence of diabetes).

■ Thrombolysis is responsible for a slightly increased risk of major bleeding, which justifies compliance with the contraindications.

■ In the **FTT collaborative group** meta-analysis, this increased risk was estimated to be 0.7% for noncerebral hemorrhage and 0.4% for hemorrhagic stroke, which essentially occurred on the day of thrombolysis or the following day. Cerebral hemorrhage has a poor prognosis, as one-half are fatal and one-quarter are responsible for stroke with moderate or severe sequelae. **Simoons** identified 3 factors predictive of intracranial hemorrhage after thrombolysis: age > 65 years, weight < 70 kg, presence of hypertension on admission.

■ Improvement of the prognosis by IV thrombolysis is directly related to the degree of coronary patency rapidly obtained.

■ This was the conclusion of the angiographic study derived from the main **GUSTO** study based on 2,431 patients with angiographic follow-up a variable time after initiation of thrombolysis (90 minutes, 180 minutes, 24 hours or 5 to 7 days). The degree of early coronary patency (90th minute) directly influenced 30-day mortality and the outcome of left ventricular function independently of the thrombolytic used (alteplase or streptokinase). Thirty-day mortality therefore did not exceed 4.4% when coronary patency was optimal (TIMI grade 3), but was 7.4% in the case of incomplete coronary patency (TIMI grade 2) and 8.9% in the case of persistent occlusion (TIMI grade 0 or 1). In parallel, preservation of left ventricular function was significantly better at the 90th minute and at the 5th-7th day in the case of early complete coronary patency compared to incomplete patency and failure of thrombolysis.

■ Alteplase is superior to streptokinase.

■ This was demonstrated by the **GUSTO** study based on more than 40,000 patients, in which accelerated alteplase infusion adapted to body weight was compared to streptokinase or a low-dose alteplase-streptokinase combination. Alteplase significantly decreased 30-day mortality (6.3% *vs* 7.3%) and the combined incidence of death or disabling stroke (6.9% *vs* 7.8%). Thus, although it increases the risk of hemorrhagic stroke, the net benefit of alteplase compared to streptokinase is 9 lives saved without disabling stroke per 1,000 patients treated.

■ Prior to the **GUSTO** study, 2 other large-scale trials, the **GISSI 2** study and the **ISIS 3** study failed to demonstrate the superiority of alteplase, used by slow infusion (over 3 or 4 hours) and without immediate heparin therapy.

■ Alteplase ensures optimal early revascularization in only about one in two patients.

■ In this same angiographic study derived from the **GUSTO** study, alteplase achieved complete coronary patency (TIMI grade 3) at the 90th minute in 54% of patients, a significantly higher proportion than that observed with streptokinase (about 30%) or the alteplase-streptokinase combination (38%).

■ The low-dose alteplase-streptokinase combination gave disappointing results.

■ Used in 10,374 patients in the **GUSTO** study, this combination compared to streptokinase alone did not decrease the 30-day mortality, but increased the risk of cerebral hemorrhage and did not modify the coronary reocclusion rate at the 5th-7th day.

■ New thrombolytics have a simplified mode of administration, but none of them have been shown to be superior to alteplase in terms of prognosis.

◆ *Three new thrombolytics, administered by a single or double IV bolus, were compared to alteplase in mortality studies.*

■ In the **GUSTO III** study conducted in 15,060 patients, reteplase did not modify the 30-day mortality (7.47% *vs* 7.24%) or the cumulative incidence of death or disabling stroke (7.89% *vs* 7.91%).

■ In the **ASSENT 2** study, which included almost 17,000 patients, tenecteplase did not modify the 30-day mortality (6.18% *vs* 6.15%), the combined incidence of death or nonfatal stroke (7.11% *vs* 7.04%) or the incidence of intracranial hemorrhage (0.93% *vs* 0.94%).

■ In the **In-TIME II** study conducted in 15,078 patients, lanoteplase did not modify mortality, but induced an excess of cerebral hemorrhage (1.13% *vs* 0.62%; p = 0.003), possibly related to excessively high-dose heparinization.

■ The combination of a GP IIb/IIIa receptor inhibitor with half-dose thrombolytic improves early coronary patency and decreases ischemic complications but with an increased bleeding risk.

■ This was the conclusion of the **GUSTO V** study conducted in 16,588 patients and the **ASSENT 3** study conducted in 6,095 patients, in which abciximab was coprescribed with either half-dose reteplase or half-dose tenecteplase.

Primary angioplasty

■ In the age of stents, thienopyridines and GP IIb/IIIa receptor inhibitors, primary angioplasty improves the prognosis of acute myocardial infarction compared to IV thrombolysis.

◆ *The superiority of conventional balloon catheter angioplasty without stenting was never clearly established.*

■ Although the meta-analysis by **Michels** based on 7 trials comprising only 1,145 patients, showed that primary angioplasty reduced mortality by 54% compared to IV thrombolysis, this superiority of conventional angioplasty was less obvious in American registries and in the **GUSTO IIb** study which included 1,138 patients.

◆ *Technical progress demonstrated the superiority of primary angioplasty over IV thrombolysis.*

■ This was the conclusion of the meta-analysis by **Keeley** based on 23 randomized trials that included 7,739 eligible patients for thrombolysis. In the short term (4 to 6 weeks), primary angioplasty decreased total mortality (7% *vs* 9%; p = 0.0002), nonfatal recurrent infarction (3% *vs* 7%; p < 0.0001), stroke (1% *vs* 2%; p = 0.0004) and the combined incidence of these events (8% *vs* 14%; p < 0.001). The significant superiority of angioplasty was maintained in the long term (6 to 18 months depending on the study) and was found to be independent of the type of thrombolytic used and possible secondary transfer of the patient for the procedure.

◆ *The time limit for angioplasty can be extended to the 12th-24th hour after onset of symptoms.*

■ This extension essentially concerns patients with severe congestive heart failure, hemodynamic or electrical instability or persistent ischemic symptoms.

◆ *Stenting in combination with thienopyridines (ticlopidine and clopidogrel) prevents acute coronary occlusion secondary to angioplasty and decreases the restenosis rate.*

■ The rationale for the ticlopidine-aspirin combination to prevent occlusive stent thrombosis has been largely demonstrated by the **ISAR 1, STARS, MATTIS and FANTASTIC** studies.

■ Clopidogrel, which has a more powerful platelet aggregation inhibitor effect, a shorter onset of action and causes fewer adverse effects, has been shown to be at least as safe and as effective as ticlopidine in the **CLASSICS** study and in the meta-analysis by **Bhatt**.

■ Stenting, compared to conventional balloon catheter angioplasty, does not modify the prognosis but decreases the repeat revascularization rate. This was the conclusion reached by the **Stent-PAMI** study based on 900 patients and one of the arms of the **CADILLAC** study that included 1,030 patients. In the meta-analysis by **Zhu** based on 9 studies and a total of 4,120 patients, stenting decreased the repeat revascularization rate by almost 60% at 6-12 months ($p < 0.001$) without modifying the mortality and with no significant reduction of the reinfarction rate ($p = 0.13$).

◆ *GP IIb/IIIa receptor inhibitors increase coronary patency and decrease early ischemic complications.*

■ Several studies, including the **SPEED** study and the **ADMIRAL** study, have shown that GP IIb/IIIa receptor inhibitors increase coronary patency prior to a dilatation procedure.

■ GP IIb/IIIa receptor inhibitors also decrease early ischemic complications by one half when they are administered before and after angioplasty, either conventional balloon catheter angioplasty without stenting, as demonstrated by the **EPIC** and **RAPPORT** studies, or combined with stenting, as demonstrated by the **ADMIRAL, ISAR 2 and ACE** studies.

■ However, this benefit was not observed in the **CADILLAC** study, in which abciximab was used at the time of angioplasty and not prior to the procedure.

■ This was also confirmed by the meta-analysis by **Montalescot** based on 6 studies comprising 931 patients, which demonstrated the superiority of early use of GP IIb/IIIa receptor inhibitors compared to administration in the catheterization suite.

■ However, the recent **FINESSE** study (see p. 112) did not demonstrate any superiority of early administration of abciximab compared to abciximab administered just before angioplasty.

■ Finally, the meta-analysis by **De Luca** based on 6 studies comprising 27,115 patients, showed that abciximab combined with primary angioplasty decreased the 30-day mortality (p = 0.047) and the reinfarction rate at 30 days (p = 0.03) and at 6 and 12 months (p = 0.01) without increasing the major bleeding risk (4.7% *vs* 4.1%).

◆ *Bivalirudin is superior to the combination of heparin and GP IIb/IIIa receptor inhibitor.*

■ This was the conclusion of the **HORIZONS-AMI** study which included 3,602 patients undergoing primary angioplasty. Bivalirudin *vs* the heparin and GP IIb/IIIa receptor inhibitor combination decreased the 30-day combined incidence of major bleeding, death, reinfarction, revascularization of the incriminated artery or stroke (9.2% *vs* 12.1%; p = 0.005) while reducing the major bleeding risk by 40% (4.9% *vs* 8.3%; p < 0.001), and reducing cardiac mortality and total mortality (2.1% *vs* 3.1%; p = 0.047). However, bivalirudin was associated with an increased risk of acute stent thrombosis during the first 24 hours.

■ The choice between IV thrombolysis and primary angioplasty must be determined case by case, taking into account the available healthcare structures and evaluation of the risk/benefit balance.

◆ *Primary angioplasty is superior to IV thrombolysis when access to the artery can be performed by an experienced team, available 24 hours a day, < 90 min after onset of IV thrombolysis, when performed.*

■ This was the conclusion of the various studies and meta-analyses that compared the two revascularization techniques.

■ However, the French **CAPTIM** study suggested that prehospital thrombolysis could be superior to primary angioplasty in patients managed during the first two hours of infarction. In this study, which included 834 patients managed by SAMU emergency teams in the first 6 hours of acute myocardial infarction and all transferred to an interventional center, primary angioplasty non-significantly decreased the combined incidence of death, reinfarction or stroke with sequelae at 30 days, compared to prehospital alteplase thrombolysis (6.2% *vs* 8.2%; p = 0.29). The efficacy of treatment in terms of prognosis was inversely correlated with the time to initiation of treatment. In 460 patients randomized in the first 2 hours after onset of symptoms, IV thrombolysis appeared to be more effective than angioplasty by decreasing the incidence of cardiogenic shock (1.3% *vs* 5.3%; p = 0.032) and 30-day mortality (2.2% *vs* 5.7%; p = 0.058).

◆ *The risk/benefit balance is in favor of angioplasty when thrombolysis is contraindicated, in the case of unstable hemodynamics and probably in the elderly, who present an increased bleeding risk related to thrombolysis.*

■ Angioplasty decreases the mortality of patients presenting a contraindication to thrombolysis by one half, as demonstrated by the American **NRMI 2, 3** and **4** registries based on almost 20,000 patients. In the group of 4,705 patients undergoing emergency angioplasty (or more rarely coronary artery bypass graft), revascularization decreased mortality by 45.8%.

■ Cardiogenic shock constitutes a good indication for emergency angioplasty, at least in subjects under the age of 75. This was demonstrated by the **SHOCK** study, which included 302 patients who developed cardiogenic shock during the first 36 hours after acute myocardial infarction. Emergency revascularization (angioplasty and/or bypass graft) compared to a conventional conservative strategy (IV thrombolysis, positive inotropic agents, intra-aortic balloon pump and assisted ventilation) non-significantly decreased hospital mortality (46.7% *vs*

56.0%; p = 0.11), but improved survival at 6 months (49.7% *vs* 36.9%; p = 0.027) and at one year (46.7% *vs* 33.6%; p < 0.03).

■ In the **GRACE** register, in 1,134 patients over the age of 70, primary angioplasty was superior to thrombolysis by decreasing the reinfarction rate by 80%, mortality by 18% and the hospital mortality or reinfarction rate by 47%.

◆ *For patients admitted to a center not equipped to perform angioplasty, the choice between thrombolysis and transfer for angioplasty essentially depends on the expected transport time.*

■ The superiority of angioplasty after transfer was reported in the **DANAMI-2** study, which included 1,572 patients, with a mean transport time of 55 minutes, and in the meta-analysis by **Zijlstra** based on 5 trials and 2,466 patients. In this analysis, primary angioplasty performed after transfer, compared to thrombolysis on the spot, significantly decreased the mortality at 4-6 weeks (6.8% *vs* 9.6%; p = 0.01) and the combined incidence of death, reinfarction or stroke (8.5% *vs* 15.5%; p < 0.001).

■ The results of facilitated angioplasty are disappointing.

■ This strategy consists of administering powerful antithrombotic therapy prior to angioplasty, comprising a low-dose thrombolytic and a GP IIb/IIIa receptor inhibitor to shorten the reperfusion time and to prevent ischemic complications related to the revascularization procedure.

■ In the meta-analysis by **Sinno**, based on 4 trials comprising a total of 725 patients, the combination of low-dose thrombolytic and GP IIb/IIIa receptor inhibitor *vs* GP IIb/IIIa receptor inhibitor alone increased the immediate complete coronary patency rate (49% *vs* 21%; p < 0.0001), but at the price of excess major bleeding (9.5% *vs* 4.7%; p = 0.007), without decreasing the 30-day mortality (3.5% *vs* 1.7%; p = 0.46) or recurrent myocardial infarction (1.1% *vs* 1.1%; p = 0.96) rates.

■ In the recent **FINESSE** study which included 2,452 patients, the combination of half-dose reteplase and abciximab, compared to early administration of abciximab and abciximab administered just before angioplasty, did not modify the combined incidence of death, ventricular fibrillation during the first 48 hours, or cardiogenic shock and congestive heart failure during the first 90 days (9.8% *vs* 10.5% *vs* 10.7%, respectively; p = 0.55), or the 90-day mortality (5.2% *vs* 5.5% *vs* 4.5%, respectively; p = 0.49).

■ Systematic early angioplasty after thrombolysis is probably beneficial, but the optimal timing of this strategy has not been clearly defined.

■ In the meta-analysis by **Collet** based on 1,508 patients, systematic angioplasty immediately following thrombolysis decreased the risk of death or reinfarction by 48% compared to a conservative strategy (deferred angioplasty reserved for recurrent ischemia).

■ However, in the recent **ASSENT 4-PCI** study, which included 1,667 patients, thrombolysis (full-dose tenecteplase) before angioplasty *vs* primary angioplasty alone (with GP IIb/IIIa receptor inhibitor in 50% of cases) induced an excess of mortality (6.0% *vs* 3.8%), reinfarction (4.1% *vs* 1.9%), thrombosis of the dilated vessel (1.9% *vs* 0.1%), reintervention on the target vessel (4.4% *vs* 1.0%), stroke (1.8% *vs* 0%) and major bleeding (5.7% *vs* 4.4%). These negative results, which led to discontinuation of the study, suggest that immediate angioplasty after thrombolysis could be harmful in the absence of powerful platelet aggregation inhibitor therapy.

■ In the **CARESS** study which included 600 patients treated in a noninterventional center by half-dose reteplase and abciximab, angioplasty immediately after transfer compared to rescue angioplasty (in the case of persistent ST-segment elevation or clinical deterioration) decreased the 30-day combined incidence of death, recurrent infarction or refractory ischemia by 60% (4.4% *vs* 10.7%; p = 0.004), without increasing the risk of major bleeding (3.4% *vs* 2.3%; p 0.47) or stroke (0.7% *vs* 1.3%; p = 0.50).

■ In the **TRANSFER-AMI** study which included 1,030 patients thrombolysed by tenecteplase, transfer for coronary angiography and angioplasty during the 6 hours following thrombolysis, compared to rescue angioplasty (associated with later coronary angiography) decreased the 30-day incidence of death, reinfarction, recurrent ischemia, heart failure or shock by 46% (10.6% *vs* 16.6%; p = 0.0013), mainly due to a reduction of recurrent ischemia without increasing major bleeding (4.6% *vs* 4.3%).

Other types of myocardial revascularization

■ Rescue angioplasty, performed immediately after failure of thrombolysis, appears to be beneficial, at least in moderately or very extensive myocardial infarction.

■ This was the conclusion of the **RESCUE** study based on only 151 patients in whom the left anterior descending artery remained occluded after IV thrombolysis. Rescue angioplasty significantly improved left ventricular function, significantly decreased the combined incidence of death and severe heart failure at the 30th day (6.4% *vs* 16.6%) and non-significantly decreased mortality (5.1% *vs* 9.6%).

■ However, in the **MERLIN** study conducted in 307 patients, rescue angioplasty did not improve 30-day survival, but decreased the repeat revascularization rate (6.5% *vs* 20.1%; p < 0.01).

■ In the **REACT** study which included 427 patients with presumed failure of thrombolysis (< 50% reduction of ST-segment elevation), rescue angioplasty *vs* repeated thrombolysis *vs* conservative management improved the 6-month survival rate free of the following events: reinfarction, stroke and heart failure (84.6% *vs* 68.7% *vs* 70.1%, respectively: p = 0.004) without modifying total mortality.

■ Finally, the meta-analysis by **Kunadian**, based on these 3 studies, suggested a globally favorable clinical benefit for rescue angioplasty which decreased mortality, reinfarction and heart failure at the price of an increased risk of stroke and bleeding.

■ Myocardial revascularization is justified in the case of recurrent ischemia after thrombolysis.

■ This was demonstrated by the **DANAMI** study, which included 1,008 thrombolysed patients who developed early recurrence of angina or positive stress test. The revascularization strategy (angioplasty or bypass graft) compared to conservative treatment, with a median follow-up of 2.4 years, decreased the rates of reinfarction (5.6% *vs* 10.5%) and unstable angina (17.9% *vs* 29.5%), without significantly modifying mortality (3.6% *vs* 4.4%).

Adjuvant therapy

Antithrombotic therapy other than thrombolysis and GP IIb/IIIa receptor inhibitors

■ Aspirin 75-160 mg daily, started as soon as possible after an IV loading dose of 250-500 mg, decreased cardiovascular mortality by 20% and this benefit is added to that provided by thrombolysis.

■ This was demonstrated by the **ISIS 2** study, which included 17,187 patients. Aspirin *vs* placebo significantly decreased mortality at the 5th week (9.4% *vs* 11.8%) and the incidence of reinfarction and nonfatal stroke. Although streptokinase decreased mortality by 23% (9.2% *vs* 12.0%), the streptokinase-aspirin combination proved to be even more effective with a 38% reduction of mortality (8.0% *vs* 13.2%).

■ Several studies have shown that a dosage of 75 to 160 mg daily is sufficient.

■ Clopidogrel must be coprescribed with aspirin.

■ This was demonstrated by the **CLARITY** study conducted in 3,491 patients ≤ 75 years, and the **COMMIT** study conducted in 45,852 patients, in whom addition of clopidogrel 75 mg daily to treatment by thrombolysis, aspirin and heparin (when justified) decreased the incidence of major cardiovascular events at 30 days, without increasing the major bleeding risk.

■ In patients over the age of 75, clopidogrel should be initiated without a loading dose.

■ Clopidogrel coprescribed with aspirin should be continued for 12 months.

■ This recommendation is based on extrapolation of the results of studies conducted in ACS without persistent ST-segment elevation (see p. 91).

■ Anticoagulant therapy for 48 hours must be coprescribed with platelet aggregation inhibitor therapy in all cases of myocardial infarction, whether or not they are reperfused.

■ In non-reperfused acute myocardial infarction, heparin decreases early morbidity and mortality and enoxaparin can replace unfractionated heparin (UFH).

■ Before the age of thrombolysis, the meta-analysis by **Collins** based on 21 small studies comprising a total of less than 6,000 patients, showed a beneficial effect of UFH during the hospital period on mortality (11.4% vs 14.9%), stroke (1.1% vs 2.1%), reinfarction (6.7% vs 8.2%) and pulmonary embolism (2.0% vs 3.8%), but with an excess of major bleeding (1.9% vs 0.9%).

■ In the **TETAMI** study, which included 1,224 patients hospitalized less than 24 hours after non-reperfused myocardial infarction, enoxaparin vs UFH non-significantly decreased the combined incidence of death, reinfarction or recurrent angina at one month (15.4% vs 17.3%), without increasing major bleeding (1.5% vs 1.3%).

■ Moderate IV heparin therapy, adapted to body weight and maintained for 48 hours, should be coprescribed with fibrin-specific thrombolytics (alteplase, tenecteplase, reteplase).

■ Several small studies have shown that UFH prevented early reocclusion related to the paradoxical prothrombotic effect observed with the use of these thrombolytic agents.

■ LMWH should replace UFH in patients under the age of 75.

■ In the **ASSENT 3** study conducted in 6,095 patients, enoxaparin combined with tenecteplase vs UFH decreased the combined incidence of death at 30 days, and reinfarction or refractory ischemia during the hospital phase (11.4% *vs* 15.4%; p = 0.0002), without increasing the bleeding risk.

■ However, the safety of use of LMWH in the elderly is uncertain.

■ In the **ASSENT-3 PLUS** study, which included 1,639 patients treated by prehospital tenecteplase thrombolysis, enoxaparin *vs* UFH increased the risk of intracranial hemorrhage (2.20% *vs* 0.97%; p = 0.047), but only in patients over the age of 75.

■ In the **CREATE** study conducted in 15,570 patients (thrombolysis in 73% and angioplasty in 6%) reviparin *vs* placebo decreased the 30-day mortality (p = 0.005) and reinfarction (p = 0.01) rates without increasing stroke, but with a slight excess of potentially fatal bleeding (0.1%).

■ In the recent **EXTRACT-TIMI 25** study which randomized 20,479 thrombolysed patients, enoxaparin continued during hospitalization compared to UFH prescribed for at least 48 hours decreased the 30-day mortality or infarction rate by 22% (9.8% *vs* 12.0%; p < 0.001) in patients thrombolysed by a fibrin-specific agent, and by 17% (10.2% *vs* 11.8%; p = 0.10) in patients thrombolysed by streptokinase. Despite an excess of major bleeding, the net benefit remained in favor of enoxaparin.

■ Fondaparinux improves the prognosis compared to UFH, particularly in patients not treated by primary angioplasty.

■ This was the conclusion of the **OASIS 6** study which included 12,092 patients. Fondaparinux prescribed for 8 days *vs* control group (UFH for 48 hours or placebo when UFH was not indicated) decreased the 30-day combined incidence of death or reinfarction (9.7% *vs* 11.2%; p = 0.008). This benefit was observed at the 9th day and at the end of the study (3 to 6 months). Fondaparinux significantly decreased mortality throughout the study. It was significantly superior *vs* placebo and *vs* UFH in thrombolysed patients (p = 0.003) and in the absence of reperfusion (p = 0.03), with a tendency to a decreased risk of severe bleeding (p = 0.13). However, it did not have any beneficial clinical effect in patients treated by primary angioplasty.

Beta-blockers

■ Before the age of coronary reperfusion, IV administration of beta-blockers decreased early morbidity and mortality.

■ This was demonstrated by the **MIAMI** study, which evaluated IV metoprolol, and especially the **ISIS 1** study. In this study, which included 16,027 patients an average of 5 hours after onset of acute myocardial infarction, atenolol 5 to 10 mg IV then orally at a dose of 100 mg daily significantly decreased vascular mortality at the 7th day by 14% with maintenance of the benefit at one year. In a retrospective analysis, the beneficial effect of the beta-blocker appeared to be related to prevention of cardiac rupture and ventricular fibrillation.

■ This efficacy of beta-blockers was confirmed in the meta-analysis by **Yusuf** based on 27 trials that included 27,000 patients, mostly at low risk. Beta-blocker therapy induced a significant 13% reduction of hospital mortality, especially during the first 2 days, a 19% reduction of nonfatal reinfarction and a 16% reduction of resuscitated cardiac arrest.

■ In the age of coronary reperfusion, beta-blockers are still indicated, even in patients with left ventricular dysfunction.

■ In the **CAPRICORN** study conducted in 1,959 patients with acute myocardial infarction and a left ventricular ejection fraction $\leq 40\%$ and treated, in one half of cases, by thrombolysis or primary angioplasty, carvedilol *vs* placebo, started between the 3rd and 21st day after hemodynamic stabilization, significantly decreased total mortality (12% *vs* 15%; p = 0.031) and nonfatal reinfarctions (3% *vs* 6%; p = 0.014) with a mean follow-up of 1.3 year.

■ However, the use IV of beta-blockers is not recommended.

■ Although the **TIMI IIB** study, which included 1,390 patients thrombolysed by alteplase, was in favor of early IV administration of beta-blockers compared to delayed oral administration, a retrospective analysis of the **GUSTO** study highlighted the potential danger of IV beta-blockers after thrombolysis, as they increased the incidence of heart failure, shock, recurrent ischemia and the need for ventricular pacing. Similarly, the meta-analysis by **Freemantle** based on 51 trials and more than 29,000 patients, did not demonstrate any benefit of early IV beta-blockers compared to oral beta-blockers.

■ In the recent **COMMIT** study conducted in 45,852 patients, IV then oral metoprolol vs placebo did not modify either the hospital mortality or the combined incidence of death, reinfarction or cardiac arrest. Although the beta-blocker decreased the risk of reinfarction (p = 0.001) and ventricular fibrillation (p = 0.01), it increased the incidence of cardiogenic shock (p < 0.00001), mainly during the first 24 hours.

Angiotensin-converting enzyme (ACE) inhibitors

■ ACE inhibitors, initiated later during hospitalization and continued longterm, very markedly improve the prognosis of myocardial infarction complicated by heart failure or left ventricular dysfunction.

■ This was demonstrated by 3 large-scale studies: the **SAVE** study, which evaluated captopril in 2,231 patients, the **AIRE** study, which evaluated ramipril in 2,006 patients and the **TRACE** study, which evaluated trandolapril in 1,749 patients.

■ In these studies, the ACE inhibitor was started at low doses, by the third day of myocardial infarction, and the dosage was gradually increased. With a mean follow-up ranging from 15 to 42 months depending on the study, the ACE inhibitor saved 42 to 74 lives per 1,000 patients treated, which represents a relative reduction of mortality of 19% to 27%. The beneficial effect of ACE inhibitors appeared to be independent of that of the other treatments administered, especially thrombolysis.

■ The value of systematic ACE inhibitor therapy in all patients by the 1st day of myocardial infarction is less apparent.

■ This was the conclusion reached by the **GISSI 3**, **ISIS 4** and **CCS 1** studies and the meta-analysis performed by the **ACE**

Inhibitor Myocardial Infarction collaborative group based on 4 studies and almost 100,000 patients. This meta-analysis showed that an ACE inhibitor started on the 1st day of myocardial infarction and continued for 4 to 6 weeks prevented 5 deaths per 1,000 patients treated and reduced the risk of heart failure.

■ In view of the risk of severe hypotension, this early prescription must be essentially reserved for patients with anterior myocardial infarction or myocardial infarction complicated by congestive heart failure, in the absence of hypotension.

Angiotensin II receptor blockers (ARBs)

■ Valsartan and candesartan can be used in myocardial infarction complicated by left ventricular dysfunction and/or heart failure, when ACE inhibitors are poorly tolerated.

■ This was demonstrated by the **VALIANT** study conducted in 14,703 patients, in which valsartan *vs* captopril, initiated during the first 10 days of acute myocardial infarction, had the same effect on two-year mortality (19.9% *vs* 19.5%).

■ The possibility of using candesartan in this indication is based on extrapolation of the favorable results of the **CHARM-Alternative** study obtained in heart failure (see p. 146).

Statins

■ Statin therapy should be systematically initiated during hospitalization at a dosage designed to achieve LDL-C < 1 g/L (2,6 mmol/L).

■ Several large-scale studies have demonstrated an improvement of the longterm prognosis when a statin was prescribed following myocardial infarction, regardless of the baseline LDL-C (see p. 43, 126).

■ However, the fact that several surveys and cohort studies have reported a largely insufficient use 6 months after myocardial infarction argues in favor of prescription of the statin during the hospital phase.

■ Other trials, currently underway, are studying the value of starting high-dose statin therapy by the 1st day of myocardial infarction in order to stabilize atheromatous plaque and consequently reduce early ischemic complications (pleiotropic effects of statins).

Nitrates

■ The efficacy of nitrates has not been demonstrated.

■ This was the conclusion reached by two large-scale studies, **GISSI 3** and **ISIS 4**, which failed to demonstrate any favorable effect of nitrates on mortality at the 5th week and thereafter. The **GISSI 3** study included nearly 19,000 patients and tested a nitrate administered from the first day of myocardial infarction by IV for 24 hours, followed by the transdermal route. The **ISIS 4** study was conducted in 58,000 patients and evaluated direct oral administration of a nitrate.

■ Similar results were reported in the **ESPRIM** study, which included 4,000 patients, in whom IV linsidomine followed by oral molsidomine did not modify the incidence of mortality or cardiac events during the hospital phase or at one year.

■ Although all of these studies are subject to criticism, it is recommended to use low-dose IV nitrates for their analgesic effects and in myocardial infarction complicated by heart failure or recurrent ischemia.

Calcium channel blockers

■ Calcium channel blockers should not be used systematically.

◆ *Overall, calcium channel blockers have not demonstrated any beneficial effect.*

■ This was the conclusion of the meta-analysis by **Held** based on 22 trials comprising about 18,000 patients randomized several hours to several days after onset of myocardial infarction. Overall, calcium channel blockers did not modify either the mortality (9.8% *vs* 9.3%) or the reinfarction rate (4.2% *vs* 4.6%).

◆ *An unfavorable tendency has even been observed with the use of first generation dihydropyridines.*

■ This was demonstrated by the **TRENT** and **SPRINT II** studies, which evaluated rapid-acting nifedipine.

■ However, no study has evaluated new generation dihydropyridines in acute myocardial infarction.

◆ *Heart-rate-lowering calcium channel blockers can be prescribed several days after myocardial infarction when beta-blockers are contraindicated and in the absence of left ventricular dysfunction.*

■ This was demonstrated by the **MDPIT** study, which evaluated diltiazem initiated between the 3rd and 15th day in 2,466 patients, and the **DAVIT II** study, which evaluated verapamil initiated between the 7th and 15th day in 1,775 patients. Varying degrees of efficacy on mortality and/or reinfarction were observed for these calcium channel blockers, but only in the absence of heart failure or left ventricular dysfunction, while these drugs had no effect or even a negative impact in the presence of these conditions.

■ In the **INTERCEPT** study conducted in 874 patients thrombolysed for a first myocardial infarction without left ventricular dysfunction, diltiazem SR 300 mg, started 36 to 96 hours after thrombolysis, almost significantly decreased the combined incidence of cardiac mortality, nonfatal reinfarction or refractory myocardial ischemia at the 6th month (23% *vs* 30%; p = 0.07), and this benefit exclusively concerned recurrent ischemia.

Other treatments

■ Lidocaine must not be used systematically for the prevention of ventricular arrhythmia during the acute phase.

■ This was the conclusion of the meta-analysis by **Mac Mahon** based on 14 studies comprising 7,165 patients. Lidocaine was responsible for a non-significant 38% increase of early mortality.

■ Systematic IV magnesium does not provide any benefit.

■ Despite the positive results of the **LIMIT 2** study, two large-scale trials permanently destroyed all hopes placed in magnesium on the basis of its potential beneficial effects (anti-ischemic, antiarrhythmic and coronary and systemic vasodilator action).

■ In the **ISIS 4** study, IV magnesium, evaluated in 58,000 patients, did not modify the mortality at 5 weeks or at 1 year, but significantly increased the incidence of heart failure, severe hypotension and episodes of bradycardia.

■ In the **MAGIC** study conducted in 6,213 high-risk patients, magnesium did not provide any benefit and did not induce any harmful effects in any of the patient subgroups analyzed.

■ Strict control of diabetes by insulin infusion is recommended during the hospital phase.

■ This was demonstrated by the **DIGAMI 1** study (see p. 75).

TIMI classification of coronary perfusion
(*Circulation* 1987; 75: 817-829)

- **Grade 0 (no perfusion):** no antegrade flow of contrast agent beyond the occlusion.

- **Grade 1 (minimal perfusion):** presence of very low antegrade flow beyond the occlusion, unable to entirely opacify the distal bed of the coronary artery.

- **Grade 2 (incomplete perfusion):** presence of antegrade flow beyond the stenosis, which entirely opacifies the distal bed of the coronary artery, but more slowly (compared to the proximal segment or other normal arteries).

- **Grade 3 (complete perfusion):** normal, non-slowed antegrade flow beyond the stenosis.

- **More simply,** grades 0 and 1 correspond to occluded coronary arteries and grades 2 and 3 correspond to patent coronary arteries, but only grade 3 reflects optimal perfusion.

Killip's Classification of heart failure during acute myocardial infarction
(Am J Cardiol 1967; 20: 457-464)

- **Class 1**   no rales or S3 gallop.
- **Class 2**   rales in the lower half of lung fields or S3 gallop.
- **Class 3**   rales in more than one half of lung fields.
- **Class 4**   cardiogenic shock.

CHAPTER 7

Post-myocardial infarction

Four basic therapeutic categories and control of risk factors

■ Except when contraindicated or poorly tolerated, 4 therapeutic categories and control of risk factors must be prescribed to all patients with myocardial infarction and therefore constitute the so-called BASIC treatment: B for beta-blockers, A for platelet aggregation inhibitors, S for statins, I for ACE inhibitors and C for control of risk factors, lifestyle changes and diet.

Beta-blockers

■ Beta-blockers significantly decrease total mortality by 20% and decrease sudden death even further.

■ In the meta-analysis by **Freemantle** based on 82 trials and 54,234 patients, beta-blockers decreased total mortality by 23% (p < 0.01) and sudden death by 43% to 51% in the 13 studies that analyzed the mode of death. They also significantly prevented the risk of reinfarction.

■ The benefit of beta-blockers persists even in the context of the modern treatment of myocardial infarction.

■ In the study by **Kernis** based on 2,442 patients treated by primary angioplasty, beta-blockers vs absence of beta-blockers decreased the 6-month mortality by 57% (p = 0.0016), and an even greater benefit was observed in patients with left ventricular dysfunction or multivessel disease.

■ Beta-blockers are even more effective in the presence of left ventricular dysfunction or heart failure.

■ This was demonstrated by the **CAPRICORN** study (see p. 118) as well as studies conducted in ischemic or nonischemic heart failure, i.e. the **US Carvedilol Heart Failure Study** and the **COPERNICUS** study which evaluated carvedilol, the **CIBIS II** study which evaluated bisoprolol and the **MERIT-HF** study conducted with metoprolol (see p. 145).

Aspirin

■ Low-dose aspirin (≤ 160 mg daily) significantly decreases total mortality and post-myocardial infarction cardiovascular mortality.

■ This was the conclusion of the **ATT** meta-analysis based on 12 studies comprising 18,788 patients, in which aspirin 75-150 mg daily decreased total mortality by 11%, cardiovascular mortality by 15%, nonfatal reinfarction by 28% and nonfatal stroke by 36%, with a mean follow-up of 2 years.

Statins

■ Statins decrease total mortality by about 20% and a target LDL-C ≤1 g/L (2,6 mmol/L) is recommended.

■ In the meta-analysis by **Larosa** based on the **4S, CARE** and **LIPID t**rials (see p. 44-46), comprising a total of 17,617 patients followed for an average of 5 to 6 years, statins significantly decreased total mortality by 23%, cardiovascular mortality by 27% and coronary mortality by 29%.

■ The **HPS** study (see p. 31, 35) confirmed that the beneficial effect of statins was independent of baseline serum cholesterol.

■ Lowering of LDL-C well below 1 g/L (2,60 mmol/L) by the prescription of high-dose statins appears to be even more beneficial.

■ In the **ALLIANCE** study conducted in 2,442 patients with stable coronary heart disease, aggressive treatment by atorvastatin titrated to lower LDL-C to below 0.8 g/L *vs* conventional management, decreased the incidence of major cardiac events by 17% (p = 0.02) with a follow-up of 4 years.

■ In the **TNT** study conducted in 10,001 patients with stable coronary heart disease with LDL-C < 1.30 g/L, atorvastatin 80 mg daily *vs* 10 mg daily more markedly lowered LDL-C (0.77 *vs* 1.01 g/L) and, with a median follow-up of 4.9 years, reduced the combined incidence of coronary mortality, nonfatal myocardial infarction, resuscitated cardiac arrest or stroke by 22% (p < 0.001) without modifying total mortality, but with an excess elevation of hepatic transaminases (1.2% *vs* 0.2%; p < 0.001).

■ In the **IDEAL** study conducted in 8,888 patients with stable coronary heart disease with a mean LDL-C of 1.24 g/L, atorvastatin 80 mg daily *vs* simvastatin 20 to 40 mg daily more markedly lowered LDL-C (0.81 g/L *vs* 1.04 g/L); with a median follow-up of 4.8 years, atorvastatin 80 mg daily tended to decrease the primary endpoint comprising coronary mortality, nonfatal infarction or resuscitated cardiac arrest by 11% (NS), but significantly decreased the incidence of nonfatal infarction (p = 0.02) and all major cardiovascular (p = 0.02) and coronary events (p < 0.001).

Angiotensin-converting enzyme (ACE) inhibitors

■ ACE inhibitors decrease total mortality, cardiovascular mortality and sudden death of post-myocardial infarction complicated by left ventricular dysfunction by about 20%.

■ In the meta-analysis by **Domanski** based on 15 studies comprising 15,104 patients, mainly the **AIRE, SAVE** and **TRACE** studies (see p. 119), ACE inhibitors significantly decreased total mortality (14.4% *vs* 16.8%), cardiovascular mortality (12.5% *vs* 14.7%) and sudden death (5.3% *vs* 6.6%).

■ The meta-analysis by **Flather** also showed that ACE inhibitors reduce recurrent myocardial infarction by 20% and rehospitalizations for heart failure by 27%.

■ ACE inhibitors prescribed on top of optimal treatment including beta-blockers, statins and aspirin remain beneficial in the absence of left ventricular dysfunction.

■ In the **HOPE** study conducted in 9,297 patients with either ischemic heart disease (80% of subjects including 53% with myocardial infarction), or a history of stroke, or peripheral artery disease, or diabetes associated with at least one other risk factor, ramipril decreased total mortality by 16%, cardiovascular mortality by 26%, myocardial infarction by 20% and stroke by 32%, with a median follow-up of 5 years.

■ In the **EUROPA** study, which included 12,218 patients with stable coronary heart disease (including 64% with a history of myocardial infarction), with a mean follow-up of 4.2 years, perindopril significantly decreased the combined incidence of cardiovascular mortality, infarction or cardiac arrest by 20% (p = 0.003) and the incidence of nonfatal infarction by 22% (p = 0.001), and tended to reduce total mortality and cardiovascular mortality. Perindopril is therefore the only ACE inhibitor with a demonstrated additive effect to that of optimal therapy comprising beta-blocker, statin and aspirin.

■ As shown by **Deckers**, the 20% risk reduction observed in overall **EUROPA** population remained constant whatever patients baseline risk level (high, medium, low). Patients at moderate-to-high risk have the most to gain in absolute and health economic terms.

■ In the **PEACE** study conducted in 8,290 patients with coronary heart disease, trandolapril was not found to have any beneficial effect on cardiovascular risk (see p. 82).

■ In the **PREAMI** study, which included 1,252 patients over the age of 65 (mean age: 72.6 years), in whom recent myocardial infarction was not complicated by left ventricular dysfunction (ejection fraction ≥ 40%; mean: 58.9%), the addition of perindopril vs placebo to optimal therapy, initiated on the 11th day at the dosage of 4 mg daily for one month then 8 mg daily for one year, decreased the risk of post-myocardial infarction ventricular remodeling, assessed on echocardiography by an increase of ventricular volume, by 46% (+ 0.7 ml vs + 4.01 ml with placebo; p < 0.001), but this beneficial action did not result in any reduction of total mortality or the number of hospitalizations for heart failure, probably because of an excessively brief follow-up. In the subgroup of patients of the **EUROPA** study presenting the same characteristics as those of the **PREAMI** study, i.e. age ≥ 65 years, history of myocardial infarction and LVEF ≥ 40%, with a mean follow-up of 4.2 years, perindopril *vs* placebo reduced the risk of major cardiac events by 36% (p = 0.03).

■ The recent meta-analyses by **Dagenais** and **Danchin** confirmed these data (see p. 82).

■ Addition of an ACE inhibitor (perindopril) to a calcium blocker in stable patients with coronary artery disease improves significantly the prognosis.

■ This was shown in a *post-hoc* analysis of **EUROPA** study by **Bertrand**: combination of perindopril and a calcium channel blocker *vs* combination of placebo and a calcium channel blocker reduced the combined incidence of cardiovascular death, myocardial infarction and resuscitated cardiac arrest by 35% (p = 0.014) and total mortality by 46% (p < 0.01). These results could be explained by a synergistic effect between perindopril and amlodipine.

Control of risk factors, lifestyle changes and diet

■ Diet improves the post-myocardial infarction prognosis.

■ In the **GISSI-Prevenzione** study, which included 11,324 patients with a mean follow-up of 3.5 years, an n-3 polyunsaturated fatty acid supplement decreased total mortality by 20%, cardiovascular mortality by 30% and sudden death by 45%.

■ In the **Lyon Diet Heart Study** conducted in 605 patients, the Mediterranean diet, rich in alpha-linolenic acid, decreased the combined incidence of cardiovascular mortality or infarction by 72% and total mortality by 66%, with a mean follow-up of 46 months.

■ Smoking cessation also improves the prognosis.

■ In the meta-analysis by **Iestra** based on the patients with coronary heart disease included in 9 cohort studies and 10 randomized trials, smoking cessation was associated with a 35% reduction of total mortality.

■ **Moderate alcohol consumption and regular physical exercise decrease total mortality.**

■ In the meta-analysis by **Iestra**, this reduction was 20% and 24%, respectively, for these two items.

■ Daily physical exercise equivalent to walking for at least 30 minutes is recommended.

■ Physical exercise, weight loss and smoking cessation contribute to increase serum HDL-C levels.

■ **The treatment of diabetes must target HbA1c < 6,5%.**

■ Although strict blood glucose control prevents small-vessel complications of diabetes, its beneficial effect on large-vessel complications has been established (see p. 56).

■ The addition of a statin to the treatment of diabetes significantly decreases the cardiovascular risk, regardless of baseline LDL-C (see p. 70-71).

■ The addition of an ACE inhibitor to the treatment of diabetes improves the cardiovascular prognosis (see p. 65-66).

■ **The treatment of hypertension must target a blood pressure < 140-90 mmHg and < 130-80 mmHg in patients with diabetes or chronic renal failure.**

■ This is the recommendation of **JNC-VII** (see p. 40).

■ Antihypertensive treatment (usually comprising 2 or 3 drugs) should preferably include an ACE inhibitor and/or a beta-blocker.

■ **High LDL-C should be treated by statins.**

■ However, a statin should also be prescribed in patients with LDL-C < 1 g/L (2.60 mmol/L).

■ Ezetimibe, a new specific inhibitor of the intestinal absorption of dietary and endogenous cholesterol, combined with a statin, provides an additional reduction of LDL-C by as much as 25%.

■ The treatment of low HDL-C (0.4 g/L i.e. 1.03 mmol/L) is not easy.

■ Physical exercise, weight loss and smoking cessation help to increase HDL-C. These measures are essential.

■ Fibrates increase HDL-C and lower triglycerides. However, their clinical efficacy remains uncertain, including in diabetic patients, who frequently have normal or below-normal LDL-C.

■ The **VA-HIT** and **BIP** studies (see p. 50) and the **DAIS** and **FIELD** studies (see p. 73) reported discordant results, mostly not significant. The efficacy of fibrates is nevertheless recognized when low HDL-C is associated with hypertriglyceridemia > 2 g/L (2.28 mmol/L) or in the case of insulin resistance. Nicotinic acid is more effective than fibrates to increase HDL-C, while decreasing triglycerides. However, no large-scale clinical trial of nicotinic acid in secondary prevention has been conducted.

■ It is reasonable to add a fibrate or nicotinic acid to statin therapy when HDL-C remains < 0.4 g/L (1.03 mmol/L) or when hypertriglyceridemia remains > 5 g/L (5.7 mmol/L) despite non-pharmacological measures.

■ This recommendation is currently not based on any large-scale randomized trial.

■ As LDL-C cannot be calculated when triglycerides are > 2 g/L, (2.28 mmol/L) treatment must target a non-LDL-C < 1.30 g/L (3.35 mmol/L).

Other drugs

Clopidogrel

■ Clopidogrel must be coprescribed with aspirin for at least 1 year after myocardial infarction.

■ This recommendation is based on extrapolation of the results of studies conducted in ACS without persistent ST-segment elevation (see p. 93-94).

■ Clopidogrel can replace aspirin when aspirin is not tolerated.

■ This was the conclusion of the **CAPRIE** study, which included 19,185 patients, 1/3 of whom had a history of myocardial infarction, 1/3 had a history of stroke and 1/3 had arterial disease of the lower limbs. Globally, clopidogrel *vs* aspirin decreased the risk of a new cardiovascular event by 8.7% (p = 0.043). The efficacy of the 2 medications was similar in the subgroup of patients with a history of myocardial infarction.

■ The value of long-term treatment with the clopidogrel-aspirin combination needs to be confirmed.

■ In the **CHARISMA** study which included 15,603 patients with either frank cardiovascular disease or multiple risk factors, the clopidogrel-aspirin combination *vs* aspirin alone, with a median follow-up of 28 months, did not modify the combined incidence of myocardial infarction, stroke or cardiovascular mortality (6.8% *vs* 7.3%; p = 0.22) which constituted the primary endpoint.

– However, although the combination appeared to be harmful in patients treated in a context of primary prevention, it was beneficial in 9,478 patients with a history of myocardial infarction or stroke or symptomatic arterial disease of the lower limbs, by significantly decreasing the primary endpoint (7.3% *vs* 8.8%; p = 0.01) without increasing the major bleeding rate (1.7% *vs* 1.5%; p = 0.50).

Anticoagulants

■ Oral anticoagulants decrease cardiovascular morbidity and mortality.

■ This was demonstrated by the **Sixty Plus Reinfarction Study**, the **WARIS** study, the **ASPECT** study and the meta-analysis by **Anand** and **Yusuf**. This meta-analysis based on 31 trials comprising 23,397 patients, showed that intense oral anticoagulation (INR 2.4-4.8) significantly decreased mortality by 22% (p < 0.001), myocardial infarction by 42% (p < 0.001) and all thromboembolic events by 63% (p < 0.001) and moderate oral anticoagulation (INR 2-3) was only very slightly less effective. However, anticoagulant therapy increases the major bleeding risk 6- to 7-fold.

■ Intense anticoagulation (INR:3-4) is more effective than aspirin only and as effective as the combination of aspirin and mild anticoagulation (INR:2-2.5).

■ This was demonstrated by the **ASPECT II** study conducted in 999 patients and the **WARIS II** study conducted in 3,630 patients.

◆ *In practice, in view of the bleeding risk and the constraints of anticoagulation, this treatment is reserved to patients not tolerating aspirin and patients with myocardial infarction associated with a high thromboembolic risk.*

Aldosterone receptor antagonists

■ Aldosterone receptor antagonists decrease total mortality and sudden death in severe heart failure and in post-myocardial infarction complicated by heart failure.

■ This was demonstrated by the **RALES** and **EPHESUS** studies which evaluated spironolactone and eplerenone, respectively (see p. 143) prescribed in combination with an ACE inhibitor and a beta-blocker.

■ The use of aldosterone receptor antagonists is contraindicated when serum potassium is > 5 mmol/L or when serum creatinine is > 250 µmol/L (28 mg/L).

■ When ACE inhibitors are not tolerated, aldosterone receptor antagonists can be coprescribed with ARBs, with the same precautions.

Angiotensin II receptor blockers (ARBs)

■ The prescription of ARBs must be considered in patients intolerant to ACE inhibitors.

■ Some ARBs can replace ACE inhibitor in myocardial infarction complicated by left ventricular dysfunction and systolic heart failure (see p. 120).

■ In the **VALIANT** study, which included 14,703 patients with myocardial infarction complicated by heart failure or with a left ventricular ejection fraction ≤ 35%, with a median follow-up of 2 years, valsartan was shown to be equivalent to captopril on total and cardiovascular mortality.

■ In the **CHARM-Alternative** study conducted in 2,028 patients with NYHA class II-III heart failure (ischemic in 2/3 of cases) and not tolerating ACE inhibitors, candesartan significantly decreased cardiovascular mortality and total mortality with a mean follow-up of 34 months.

■ The addition of an ARB to an ACE inhibitor further reduced cardiovascular mortality in patients with heart failure.

■ This was demonstrated by the **VAL-HeFT** and **CHARM-Added** studies (see p. 147).

■ As for ACE inhibitors, treatment should be initiated at a low dosage, when possible after reducing the dose of diuretics, and should then be gradually increased until the optimal dose used in clinical trials while regularly monitoring serum creatinine and serum potassium. A 10% to 15% elevation of serum creatinine is acceptable. In the absence of heart failure, telmisartan is equivalent to an ACE inhibitor (ramipril), but coprescription of the two drugs is not recommended.

■ This is the conclusion of the recent **ONTARGET** (see p. 25).

Nitrates

■ The long-term value of nitrates has not been studied.

■ Nitrates, prescribed for 5 to 6 weeks in the **GISSI 3** and **ISIS 4** studies (see p. 121) did not demonstrate any marked benefit.

■ However, they remain useful in patients with residual angina and possibly in heart failure.

Calcium channel blockers

■ Verapamil can be prescribed when beta-blockers are poorly tolerated, in the absence of heart failure.

■ This was the conclusion of the **DAVIT II** study (see p. 122), the **CRIS** study, in which the benefit was not significant, and the **INVEST** study conducted in 6,391 hypertensive patients with coronary heart disease, 1/3 of whom had a history of myocardial infarction, in whom the verapamil SR-trandolapril combination was found to be as effective as the atenolol-hydrochlorothiazide combination in the prevention of cardiovascular morbidity and mortality.

■ Diltiazem and new generation dihydropyridines can be prescribed in patients with residual angina or hypertension.

■ Diltiazem prescribed in the absence of left ventricular dysfunction was shown to be effective on ischemic complications in the **MDPIT** and **INTERCEPT** studies (see p. 122).

■ Amlodipine and felodipine, which have not been specifically studied in post-myocardial infarction, are well tolerated in chronic heart failure, as demonstrated by the **PRAISE 1** and **2** and **VHeFT III** studies (see p. 151).

Antiarrhythmic drugs (apart from beta-blockers)

■ Class I antiarrhythmics increase the mortality and must be avoided, especially in patients with left ventricular dysfunction.

■ This was the conclusion of the **CAST I** and **CAST II** studies conducted with encainide, flecainide or moricizine, and the meta-analysis by **Teo**.

■ Amiodarone decreases sudden death after myocardial infarction and can be used in patients with left ventricular dysfunction, but has little or no effect on total mortality and its extracardiac adverse effects limit its long-term use.

■ This was demonstrated by the **EMIAT** study conducted in 1,486 patients with myocardial infarction complicated by heart failure, and the **CAMIAT** study, which included 1,202 patients with myocardial infarction associated with premature ventricular complexes.

■In the **ATMA** meta-analysis based on 13 trials and 6,553 patients with myocardial infarction or heart failure, amiodarone decreased total mortality by 13% (p = 0.030) and sudden death by 29% (p = 0.03).

■The **ECMA** meta-analysis based on the **EMIAT** and **CAMIAT** studies, showed that the beneficial effect of amiodarone was particularly marked in patients already treated with beta-blockers.

Implantable cardioverter-defibrillator (ICD)

■ In secondary prevention, ICD improves the prognosis *vs* amiodarone and must represent first-line treatment.

■Secondary prevention is indicated in patients surviving cardiac arrest due to ventricular tachycardia-fibrillation and those with poorly supported sustained ventricular arrhythmia.

■ The meta-analysis by **Connolly** based on the **CASH, AVID** and **CIDS** studies, showed that ICD *vs* amiodarone significantly decreased total mortality by 28% and sudden death by 50% with a mean follow-up of 2.3 years. However, the superiority of ICD was only observed when the left ventricular ejection fraction was ≤ 35%.

■ In primary prevention (absence of potentially fatal sustained ventricular arrhythmia), ICD decreases post-myocardial infarction mortality by one half in the presence of left ventricular dysfunction (LVEF < 40%), asymptomatic unsustained ventricular tachycardia (VT) and inducible VT.

■This was demonstrated by the **MADIT I** study, which included 196 patients and the **MUSTT** study conducted in 704 patients.

■ In primary prevention (absence of potentially fatal sustained ventricular arrhythmia), asymptomatic severe (LVEF < 30%) left ventricular dysfunction or LVEF ≤ 35% with NYHA class II or III heart failure constitute indications for ICD.

■ This was shown by the **MADIT II** study, which included 1,232 patients with a LVEF ≤ 30% at least one month after myocardial infarction, ICD significantly decreased total mortality by 31% with a mean follow-up of 20 months.

■ This was demonstrated by the **SCD-HeFT** study, which included 2,521 patients with NYHA class II-III heart failure (ischemic in one half of cases) and a LVEF ≤ 35%. With a mean follow-up of 46 months, ICD *vs* placebo decreased total mortality by 23% (p = 0.007), while amiodarone had no significant effect.

Antiarrhythmics – Vaughan-Williams' classification
(*J Clin Pharmacol* 1984;24:129-138) [modified by including new molecules]

- **Class I**   Depression of the rapid sodium channel
  - **Ia**   intermediate kinetics and depression of the potassium channel (prolong repolarization)
quinidine, procainamide, disopyramide, ajmaline
  - **Ib**   rapid kinetics lidocaine, mexiletine, diphenylhydantoin, tocainide
  - **Ic**   slow kinetics, flecainide, encainide, propafenone, lorcainide, moricizine, cibenzoline

- **Class II**   Beta-adrenergic blockade
  - beta-blockers

- **Class III**   Potassium channel blockade (prolong repolarization)

- **Class IV**   Calcium channel blockade
  - verapamil, diltiazem, bepridil

CHAPTER 8

Chronic heart failure

Prevention

■ The development of heart failure can be prevented or delayed with early treatment of diseases that ultimately lead to heart failure, especially hypertension and coronary heart disease.[1]

■ In practice, this implies rigorous management of patients at high cardiovascular risk.

Non-pharmacological treatment

Sodium restriction

■ Strict reduction of sodium intake is especially recommended in advanced heart failure.

■ Replacement salts must be used cautiously because they often contain potassium and a high consumption could lead to hyperkalemia, especially when they are associated with an ACE inhibitor and/or aldosterone receptor inhibitor.

---

1 Statements developed in this chapter are based on Recommendations published by the ESC (2005).

Physical training

■ Far from being contraindicated, physical training is recommended in the treatment of chronic heart failure, especially in patients with the lowest exercise tolerance.

■ Heart failure is known to induce progressive deterioration of functional capacity, accentuated by a sedentary lifestyle.

■ Controlled studies have shown that regular moderate physical training:

– improves symptoms in patients with stable chronic heart failure (class NYHA II-III);

– modifies the peripheral circulation, increases the aerobic capacity, delays activation of anaerobic metabolism, lowers sympathetic tone and increases vagal tone;

– has a more uncertain effect on the left ventricular ejection fraction and on morbidity and mortality.

■ According to the **ExTra MATCH** meta-analysis based on 9 prospective studies comprising 801 patients with a mean follow-up of 729 days, physical exercise compared to the control group decreased mortality by 35% ($p = 0.015$).

■ However, in the **HF-ACTION** study (*AHA Congress*, 2008) conducted in 2,331 patients with NYHA class II-IV chronic heart failure (mean LVEF: 25%), with a mean follow-up of 2.5 years, regular cardiac retraining prescribed on top of usual care was safe but did not significantly decrease the incidence of the primary endpoint comprising all-cause death and all-cause hospitalization (HR 0.93; $p = 0.13$).

Pharmacological treatment

Angiotensin-converting enzyme (ACE) inhibitors

■ ACE inhibitors, mixed venous and arterial vasodilators, improve survival, symptoms, functional capacity and reduce the number of hospitalizations at all stages of heart failure.

■ This was demonstrated for the first time by the CONSENSUS study in severe heart failure (NYHA class IV; LVEF < 30%): the addition of enalapril to conventional treatment (target dosage: 40 mg daily) *vs* placebo decreased mortality by 40% at 6 months (p = 0.002) and 31% at 12 months (p = 0.001).

■ This was demonstrated by the treatment arm of the SOLVD study and the VHeFT II study, also conducted with enalapril *vs* placebo in patients with mild-to-moderate heart failure (NYHA class II-III; LVEF respectively ≤ 35% and < 45%).

■ This was demonstrated by the prevention arm of the SOLVD study conducted in 4,228 patients with isolated left ventricular dysfunction, with no signs of heart failure (NYHA class I-II; LVEF ≤ 35%) in whom, with a mean follow-up of 37.4 months, enalapril (target dosage: 20 mg daily) *vs* placebo significantly reduced the number of deaths or hospitalizations for heart failure by 20% (p < 0.001). This was also demonstrated by the SAVE study conducted in 2,231 patients with acute myocardial infarction and a mean LVEF of 31% in the absence of clinical signs of heart failure; with a mean follow-up of 42 months, captopril (target dosage: 150 mg daily) *vs* placebo significantly decreased total mortality by 19% (p = 0.019) and cardiovascular mortality by 21% (p = 0.014).

■ Consequently, ACE inhibitors must be prescribed very extensively as first-line treatment to all patients with left ventricular dysfunction (left ventricular ejection fraction < 40-45%), whether or not they are symptomatic.

■ The meta-analyses by **Garg and Yusuf** and **Shekelle** showed that the relative reduction of mortality and the number of hospitalizations for heart failure was observed independently of age, gender, NYHA functional class and etiology of heart disease.

■ However, ACE inhibitors appear to be less effective in black subjects; in **Exner's** retrospective analysis of the SOLVD study, enalapril 2.5-20 mg daily *vs* placebo reduced the hospitalization rate for heart failure in white patients by 44%, but did not significantly decrease the hospitalization rate in black patients (p = 0.74), with a mean follow-up of 34 months.

■ ACE inhibitors are not interchangeable.

■ Only 6 of the 10 ACE inhibitors available in the USA significantly improve survival and reduce the morbidity of patients with heart failure or myocardial infarction: captopril (**ISIS 4** study), enalapril (**CONSENSUS** and **SOLVD** studies), lisinopril (**GISSI 3** study), ramipril (**AIRE** and **HOPE** studies), trandolapril (**TRACE** study), perindopril (**EUROPA** study).

■ It is unknown whether the other 4 ACE inhibitors (benazepril, fosinopril, moexipril, equinapril) have similar effects in these indications.

Thiazide and loop diuretics

■ Diuretics represent the essential treatment for congestive heart failure responsible for peripheral edema or pulmonary overload.

■ When prescribed in this setting, diuretics rapidly improve breathlessness and exercise tolerance. However, no randomized trial has evaluated their effect on mortality.

■ Loop diuretics are usually used as they are the most effective.

■ At equivalent dosages, all diuretics of this class increase diuresis to a comparable degree.

■ Thiazide diuretics are much less effective than loop diuretics.

■ This is especially the case when glomerular filtration rate is < 30 ml/min, a situation frequently observed in elderly patients with heart failure.

■ Thiazide diuretics can be coprescribed with loop diuretics in severe heart failure.

■ These two therapeutic categories have a synergistic action. According to the randomized trial by **Channer**, this combination is probably more effective than an increased dosage of loop diuretics.

■ Long-term loop diuretic therapy increases the risk of arrhythmic death.

■This was demonstrated by the retrospective studies conducted by **Cooper** on data from the **SOLVD** study (see p. 141) and **Neuberg** on data from the **PRAISE 1** study (see p. 151).

◆ *In contrast, also according to **Cooper**, potassium-sparing diuretics, alone or in combination with a potassium-lowering diuretic, are not accompanied by an increased relative risk of arrhythmic death (RR: 0.90; p = 0.6).*

Aldosterone receptor blockers

■Aldosterone can have harmful effects by promoting myocardial and vascular fibrosis, potassium and magnesium depletion, activation of the sympathetic nervous system, inhibition of the parasympathetic nervous system and baroreceptor dysfunction. ACE inhibitors do not sufficiently reduce circulating aldosterone levels.

■Aldosterone receptor blockers, in combination with ACE inhibitors, beta-blockers and diuretics, are recommended in patients with advanced heart failure (class NYHA III-IV) to improve survival and morbidity.

■ Aldosterone receptor blockers, in combination with ACE inhibitors and beta-blockers, are recommended in left ventricular systolic dysfunction related to myocardial infarction, accompanied by signs of heart failure or diabetes, to reduce mortality and morbidity.

■This was demonstrated by the **RALES** study conducted in 1,663 patients with severe heart failure (NYHA class III-IV; LVEF ≤ 35%). With a mean follow-up of 24 months, spironolactone 25-50 mg daily (mean dose: 26 mg daily) *vs* placebo, prescribed in addition to standard therapy (ACE inhibitor, furosemide, or even cardiac glycosides) significantly decreased the relative risk of total mortality by 30% (p < 0.001), due to a 36% reduction of the relative risk of death from progressive heart failure (p < 0.001) and a 29% reduction of the relative risk of cardiac sudden death (p = 0.02).

■This was also demonstrated by the **EPHESUS** study conducted in 6,632 patients with LVEF ≤ 40% and signs of heart failure, included 3 to 14 days after acute myocardial infarction; with a mean follow-up of 16 months, the addition of eplerenone (mean dosage: 43 mg daily) *vs* placebo decreased total mortality by 15% (p = 0.008) and cardiovascular mortality by 17% (p = 0.005).

Beta-blockers

■ For a long time, beta-blockers were formally contraindicated in heart failure, especially because of their negative inotropic effects. We now know that left ventricular dysfunction stimulates neuroendocrine systems, including the sympathetic nervous system, creating, in the long term, a harmful situation which worsens heart failure.

■ The paradox of the prescription of beta-blockers in heart failure is therefore only apparent. However, in practice, treatment must be instituted cautiously in stabilized patients, i.e. in the absence of an acute episode of heart failure, by starting with a low dose that is gradually increased (titration period).

■ In the absence of a contraindication, beta-blockers must be prescribed to all patients with chronic heart failure (NYHA class II-IV) regardless of its stage and its etiology (ischemic or nonischemic) .

◆ *Beta-blockers associated with ACE inhibitors and diuretics reduce morbidity, the global hospitalization rate, especially hospitalizations for acute episodes of heart failure; they increase the left ventricular ejection fraction, improve the NYHA functional class and slow the progression of heart failure.*

■ This beneficial effect is regularly observed independently of age, gender, functional class, left ventricular ejection fraction, and the etiology of the heart disease.

■ This was demonstrated at the beginning of the 1990s by two large-scale randomized studies, **MDC** and **CIBIS I**, although neither of them demonstrated a reduction of mortality with beta-blockers.

◆ *Beta-blockers significantly reduce the mortality of chronic heart failure.*

■ This was demonstrated for the first time in 1999, by two large-scale randomized studies **CIBIS II** and **MERIT-HF**.

■ In the **CIBIS II** study conducted in 2,647 patients with NYHA class III-IV chronic heart failure (mean LVEF: 26.6%) with a mean follow-up of 1.3 year, addition of bisoprolol (target dosage: 10 mg daily) *vs* placebo to conventional therapy decreased the relative risk of all-cause mortality by 34% (p = 0.0001) and the relative risk of sudden death by 44% (p = 0.0011).

■ In the **MERIT-HF** study conducted in 3,991 patients with NYHA class II-III heart failure (mean LVEF: 28%) with a follow-up of 1 year, addition of metoprolol (target dosage: 200 mg daily) *vs* placebo to conventional therapy significantly reduced the relative risk of total mortality by 34% (p = 0.00009) and the relative risk of sudden death by 41% (p = 0.0002).

■ Almost at the same time, the **US Carvedilol Heart Failure** study conducted with carvedilol (target dosage: 50 mg daily), a new generation beta-blocker with alpha-blocker properties and therefore vasodilator, antioxidant and antiproliferative effects, reached the same conclusion in mild heart failure, mild-to-moderate heart failure (**MOCHA** study, **PRECISE** study, **ANZ-HeFT** study) and severe heart failure, as in the **COPERNICUS** study conducted in 2,289 patients (mean LVEF: 19.8% ± 4.0%).

■ The **COMET** study showed that carvedilol could even be superior to metoprolol.

■ Beta-blocker therapy is effective even in the elderly.

■ In the **SENIORS** study conducted in 2,128 patients over the age of 70 years (mean age: 76 years), with a follow-up of 21 months, the addition of nebivolol 5 to 10 mg daily vs placebo to optimal therapy decreased the incidence of the composite endpoint comprising total mortality and hospitalization for cardiovascular disease by 14% (p = 0.039).

■ Beta-blockers are also the only antiarrhythmics which significantly decrease total mortality and sudden death in patients with heart failure.

■ Consequently, whenever they are well tolerated, beta-blockers have a favorable effect on unsustained ventricular arrhythmias supported. In the **CIBIS II** study, bisoprolol decreased the relative risk of death by 34% (p < 0.0001), due to a 44% reduction of sudden death. In the **MERIT-HF** study, metoprolol significantly reduced the relative risk of all-cause mortality by 34% (p = 0.0009) and the relative risk of sudden death by 41% (p = 0.0002). Studies performed with carvedilol reported globally similar results.

■ The various beta-blockers are not interchangeable.

　■ Consequently, only beta-blockers whose efficacy has been demonstrated in large-scale clinical trials should be used in the treatment of chronic heart failure, i.e. bisoprolol, carvedilol, metoprolol (succinate) and nebivolol.

■ The prescription of beta-blockers in chronic heart failure is still very insufficient.

　■ According to the results of the **Euro Heart Failure** survey conducted in 11,304 patients with chronic heart failure evaluated for 6 weeks in 115 hospitals in 24 countries, only 36.9% of patients were treated with a beta-blocker and only 17.2% of them received triple therapy comprising diuretics, ACE inhibitors and beta-blockers.

Angiotensin II receptor blockers (ARBs)

■ When ACE inhibitors are contraindicated or poorly tolerated, ARBs represent a therapeutic alternative, which reduces cardiovascular morbidity and mortality.

　■ This was demonstrated by the **VALIANT** study (see p. 120, 134).

　■ This was confirmed by the **CHARM-Alternative** study conducted in 2,028 patients with chronic heart failure (essentially NYHA class II-III; mean LVEF: 30%) not supporting ACE inhibitor therapy. Addition of candesartan 4 to 8 mg daily *vs* placebo to optimal therapy decreased the relative risk of the primary composite endpoint (cardiovascular mortality or hospitalizations for heart failure) and each of its components by 23% (p < 0.0001), with a mean follow-up of 33.7 months.

♦ *Improvement of survival is due to a reduction of sudden death and death due to deterioration of heart failure.*

■ In the **CHARM** program, comprising the **CHARM-Alternative, CHARM-Added** and **CHARM-Preserved** studies with a total of 7,599 patients, candesartan reduced the risk of sudden death by 15% (p = 0.036) and the risk of death due to deterioration of heart failure by 22% (p = 0.008). This beneficial effect was more marked when left ventricular ejection fraction was 40%.

■ An ARB can be coprescribed with an ACE inhibitor when patients remain symptomatic.

■ This was demonstrated by the **VAL-HeFT** study conducted in 5,010 patients with chronic heart failure (essentially NYHA class II-III; LVEF < 40%), in whom addition of valsartan 160 mg x 2 daily *vs* placebo to conventional therapy, comprising an ACE inhibitor in 93% of cases, did not modify total mortality (primary endpoint) but significantly reduced the other primary composite morbidity and mortality endpoint by 13.2%, essentially due to a significant 27.5% reduction (p = 0.001) of the number of hospitalizations for heart failure.

– Combined therapy was generally well tolerated. The adverse events leading to discontinuation included dizziness (in 1.6% of the patients in the valsartan group and 0.4% of those in the placebo group; p < 0.001), hypotension (1.3% and 0.8%, respectively; p = 0.124) and renal impairment (1.1% and 0.2%; p < 0.001).

■ This was confirmed by the **CHARM-Added** study conducted in 2,548 patients with chronic heart failure (essentially NYHA class II-III; mean LVEF: 28%), in whom addition of candesartan (target dose: 32 mg daily) *vs* placebo to optimal therapy, which always comprised an ACE inhibitor, decreased the relative risk of the main composite endpoint (cardiovascular mortality or hospitalization for heart failure) by 15% (p = 0.010).

– These benefits were obtained at the expense of infrequent side effects. The adverse events leading to discontinuation included: hypotension (in 4.5% of the patients in the candesartan group and in 3.1% of those in the placebo group; p = 0.079), increase in creatinine (7.8% and 4.1% respectively; p = 0.0001), hyperkalemia (3.4% and 0.7%; p < 0.0001).

■ ARBs can be safely coprescribed with beta-blockers, either alone or in combination with an ACE inhibitor.

■ Some studies, such as the **ELITE II** and **VAL-HeFT** studies, showed that the losartan-beta-blocker or valsartan-beta-blocker-ACE inhibitor combination tended to increase the incidence of the combined morbidity and mortality end-point, raising the question of whether intense blockade of multiple neuroendocrine systems induced by concomitant treatment with an ARB and a beta-blocker could be harmful in patients with heart failure.

■ This is not the case, as this negative impact was not observed in three recent large-scale clinical trials: **OPTIMAAL** conducted in post-myocardial infarction with the losartan-beta-blocker combination, **CHARM-Added** conducted in chronic heart failure with the candesartan-beta-blocker combination and **VALIANT** study conducted with the valsartan-captopril-beta-blocker combination in acute myocardial infarction complicated by left ventricular dysfunction or heart failure.

Positive inotropic agents

Digoxin

■ Digoxin does not modify total mortality, but significantly reduces the combined risk of hospitalization and death due to deterioration of heart failure.

■ This was demonstrated by the **DIG** study conducted in 6,800 patients with chronic heart failure (mostly NYHA class II-III) in sinus rhythm. With a follow-up of 4 years, digoxin 0.125-0.50 mg daily *vs* placebo in addition to an ACE inhibitor and diuretics, did not modify total mortality but significantly decreased the relative risk of the combined incidence of death and hospitalizations for heart failure by 25% (p < 0.001).

■ However, this result was achieved at the price of a 14% increase of the relative risk of death from arrhythmia or coronary heart disease (p = 0.04).

◆ *In practice, digoxin can be used in patients with chronic heart failure in sinus rhythm when symptoms persist despite well conducted therapy.*

■ Contrary to previous recommendations, digoxin must be prescribed at a low dosage to obtain plasma digoxin levels of about 0.5 to 0.9 ng/mL.

■ This was demonstrated by **Adams'** study based on data from the **PROVED** and **RADIANCE** studies and the retrospective analysis by **Rathore** based on the data of 3,782 male patients included in the **DIG** study.

◆ *At these low concentrations, the neuroendocrine effect of digoxin outweighs its hemodynamic effects.*

■ Digoxin is indicated in atrial fibrillation accompanied by even minor signs of heart failure.

■ In this situation, the cardiotonic slows the resting ventricular rate by a vagotonic effect on the atrioventricular node, but appears to be less effective on ventricular rate on exertion and has no effect on control of paroxysmal atrial fibrillation.

■ The dosage can be higher in this indication, but serum digoxin levels must not exceed 2 ng/mL. According to **Farshi**, only the digoxin-atenolol combination has a demonstrated efficacy on control of ventricular rate.

Other positive inotropic agents

■ The long-term prescription of other positive inotropic agents is not recommended, as they increase mortality.

◆ *This is the case for long-term weekly IV dobutamine infusion.*

■ Dobutamine, used to correct hemodynamic disturbances associated with acute episodes of heart failure, can be responsible for tachyphylaxis, increased heart rate, serious arrhythmia and/or myocardial ischemia (**DICE** study).

■ Dobutamine is also less effective in the presence of concomitant beta-blocker therapy, as it acts via stimulation of beta-adrenergic receptors.

◆ *This is the case for sympathomimetics.*

■ Sympathomimetics activate cyclic AMP synthesis by stimulating myocardial beta-1adrenergic receptors (prenalterol, L-dopa, xamoterol, ibopamine) or vascular beta-2 adrenergic receptors, which are also responsible for arterial vasodilatation (salbutamol, terbutaline, pirbuterol).

■ In the **PRIME II** study conducted in 1,906 patients with severe heart failure (NYHA class III-IV), with a follow-up of about one year, addition of oral ibopamine 300 mg daily *vs* placebo to optimal conventional treatment significantly increased the relative risk of mortality by 26% (p = 0.017).

◆ *This is the case for phosphodiesterase inhibitors.*

■ They prolong the action of cyclic AMP (c AMP) by inhibiting phosphodiesterase, the enzyme responsible for breakdown of cAMP (amrinone, enoximone, milrinone, pimobendan, vesnarinone) and they exert both inotropic and vasodilator effects.

■ Although they improve short-term symptoms and signs of heart failure (as demonstrated by the **WEST** study), long-term prescription is not recommended as their efficacy tends to wane with time due to desensitization of beta-adrenergic receptors, and they increase mortality (as demonstrated by the **PROMISE, PICO** and **VEST** studies conducted with oral milrinone, pimobendan, and vesnarinone, respectively).

Vasodilators

■ Since publication of the **VHeFT I** study, vasodilator therapy is an integral part of the treatment of heart failure. In particular, vasodilators counteract peripheral vasoconstriction secondary to sympathetic nervous system and renin-angiotensin-aldosterone system hyperactivity, which is a constant feature of left ventricular dysfunction.

■ Vasodilators with a direct action comprise: venous vasodilators (nitrates, molsidomine), arterial vasodilators (dihydralazine, dihydropyridines), which induce arterial and secondarily venous smooth muscle relaxation, which decreases left ventricular outflow resistance and increases the venous reservoir capacitance. Vasodilators with a direct action do not have a specific role in the treatment of heart failure, but they can be used as adjuvant therapy.

■ The hydralazine-nitrate combination may be justified in patients not tolerating ACE inhibitors and ARBs.

■ The hydralazine-nitrate combination was the first vasodilator treatment shown to improve the prognosis of mild-to-moderate chronic heart failure.

■ In the **VHeFT I** study conducted in 642 patients with mild-to-moderate chronic heart failure (NYHA class II-III; left ventricular ejection fraction < 45%), addition of hydralazine 300 mg daily and isosorbide dinitrate 160 mg daily *vs* placebo to treatment with digoxin and diuretics significantly decreased (p < 0.028) mortality by 34% at 2 years and 36% at 3 years, but did not modify the incidence of hospitalizations for heart failure.

■ This was also demonstrated by the **AAHeFT** study conducted in 1,050 black patients with moderate-to-severe heart failure (NYHA class II-IV; left ventricular ejection fraction < 30%), in whom addition of a fixed dose of one capsule then two capsules of hydralazine 37.5 mg-isosorbide dinitrate 20 mg tid *vs* placebo to optimal therapy significantly reduced total mortality by 43% (p = 0.01) and the number of hospitalizations for heart failure by 33% (p = 0.001) and improved quality of life scores (p = 0.02), with a follow-up of 18 months.

■ Nitrates can be used as adjuvant therapy in the case of angina or persistent dyspnea.

■ No therapeutic trial in heart failure has yet been designed to evaluate the impact of nitrates on mortality.

Calcium channel blockers

■ New generation dihydropyridines (amlodipine and felodipine) have a neutral effect on survival.

■ This was demonstrated by the combined analysis of the **PRAISE 1** and **2** studies conducted with amlodipine.

■ This was confirmed by the **VHeFT III** study, in which addition of felodipine 5-10 mg daily *vs* placebo to conventional treatment, with a mean follow-up of 18 months, did not modify either mortality or the hospitalization rate, but prevented deterioration of exercise tolerance and quality of life.

◆ *This effect can be useful in angina and/or HT associated with heart failure, which can therefore be treated by this therapeutic category.*

Antithrombotics

■ Anticoagulant therapy is formally indicated when heart failure is associated with a high thromboembolic risk.

■ This is the case in the presence of advanced heart failure (marked reduction of left ventricular ejection fraction and cardiac dilatation), rheumatic heart disease, especially mitral valve disease, atrial fibrillation, mobile left ventricular thrombus, or a history of thromboembolism.

■ During anticoagulant therapy, the annual bleeding rate is about 5% to 6% and the fatal hemorrhage rate is about 0.8%.

■ The bleeding risk increases markedly with age, comorbidity, and drug interactions and elderly patients with a high embolic risk are at greatest risk of bleeding complications of anticoagulant therapy.

Antiarrhythmics

Class I antiarrhythmics

■ Class I antiarrhythmics must not be used in patients with chronic heart failure, as they decrease survival.

■ Since publication of the **CAST I** and **II** studies, it is known that class I anti-arrhythmics (encainide, flecainide, moricizine) increase total mortality and sudden death due to their negative inotropic and proarrhythmic effects, as they can induce fatal ventricular arrhythmia.

Class II antiarrhythmics

■ Beta-blockers are the only antiarrhythmics which significantly decrease sudden death in patients with chronic heart failure.

■ Whenever they are well tolerated, beta-blockers therefore have a favorable effect on unsustained ventricular arrhythmias in patients with heart failure.

■ In the **CIBIS II study** conducted in 2,647 patients with chronic heart failure (NYHA class III [83%]-IV [17%]) with a mean follow-up of 1.3 year, bisoprolol 1.25-10 mg daily *vs* placebo significantly decreased the relative risk of death by 34% (p < 0.0001) due to a 44% reduction of sudden death.

■ In the **MERIT-HF** study conducted in 3,991 patients with chronic heart failure (NYHA class II [41%]-III [56%]) with a mean follow-up of 1.3 year, metoprolol CR/XL 12.5-200 mg daily *vs* placebo significantly reduced the relative risk of all-cause mortality by 34% (p = 0.0009) and the relative risk of sudden death by 41% (p = 0.0002).

■ Studies conducted with carvedilol indicate globally similar results.

Class III antiarrhythmics

■ Amiodarone is effective on most supraventricular and ventricular arrhythmias.

  ■ Amiodarone can restore and maintain sinus rhythm in patients with heart failure and atrial fibrillation; it can also improve the electrical cardioversion success rate.

  ■ Amiodarone is the only antiarrhythmic devoid of any clinically perceptible negative inotropic effects.

■ However, routine use of amiodarone is not indicated in heart failure because it does not reduce total mortality and is not devoid of adverse effects.

  ■ In the **STAT-CHF** study conducted in 674 patients with chronic heart failure (NYHA class III-IV; left ventricular ejection fraction ≤ 40%), presenting ventricular arrhythmias (at least 10 asymptomatic premature ventricular complexes per hour), amiodarone 300 mg daily *vs* placebo did not significantly modify total mortality and sudden death, with a mean follow-up of 45 months.

  ■ In the **SCD-HeFT** study (see p. 160) conducted in 2,521 patients with chronic heart failure (NYHA class II-III;

LVEF ≤ 35%) with a mean follow-up of 46 months, amiodarone 800 mg daily for one week, then 400, 300 or 200 mg daily according to body weight > 90.9 kg, between 68.2 and 90.9 kg or < 68.2 kg, did not modify mortality and did not appear to be any more effective than placebo, while ICD *vs* placebo decreased total mortality by 23% (p = 0.007).

■ Dronedarone, an amiodarone analog, but with less thyroid toxicity, is currently being evaluated in patients with chronic heart failure.

■ In the **ATHENA** study conducted in 4,628 patients with intermediate- or high-risk atrial fibrillation/flutter, i.e. age 75 ≥ years or ≥ 70 years in the presence of stroke or TIA, left atrial hypertrophy, left ventricular ejection fraction < 40%, 29% of whom had a history of heart failure, the addition of dronedarone 400 mg twice daily to standard therapy comprising beta-blockers, calcium channel blockers, ACE inhibitors, ARBs, digoxin, statins and oral anticoagulants *vs* placebo and with a mean follow-up of 21 months increased the time to onset of the first event of the primary composite endpoint, i.e. hospitalization for cardiovascular disease or all-cause mortality, by 24% (p < 0.001), decreased cardiovascular mortality by 29% (p = 0.034), stroke by 34% (p = 0.027) hospitalizations for cardiovascular disease by 25% (p < 0.001) and arrhythmic deaths by 45% (p = 0.01).

Statins

■ Statins do not significantly improve survival of patients with chronic heart failure.

■ This was demonstrated by the **CORONA** study conducted in 5,000 patients with a mean age of 72.6 ± 7.1 years with ischemic systolic heart failure (mean left ventricular ejection fraction: 31%) in whom addition of rosuvastatin 10 mg daily *vs* placebo to standard therapy tended to decrease the incidence of the primary endpoint comprising cardiovascular mortality, myocardial infarction or nonfatal stroke by 8% (p = 0.12; NS) with a follow-up of 33 months, but did not modify either total mortality or cardiovascular mortality. In contrast, it significantly decreased the all-cause hospitalization rate (p = 0.007) and the cardiovascular hospitalization rate (p < 0.001), especially for heart failure (p < 0.01).

■ This was confirmed by the **GISSI 3 HF** study conducted in 4,574 patients with a mean age of 68 ± 11 years with chronic heart failure (NYHA class II-IV) irrespective of cause and left ventricular ejection fraction; with a median follow-up of 3.9 years, addition of rosuvastatin 10 mg daily *vs* placebo to optimal heart failure therapy did not modify the incidence of the primary composite endpoint (time to death and time to death or admission to hospital for cardiovascular reasons).

Omega-3 polyunsaturated fatty acids

■ Omega-3 polyunsaturated fatty acid supplementation slightly decreases the mortality of patients with chronic heart failure.

■ This was demonstrated by the **GISSI 3 HF** study conducted in 6,975 patients with a mean age of 67 ± 11 years with NYHA class II-IV heart failure, hospitalized for chronic heart failure during the previous year. With a median follow-up of 3.9 years, addition of n-3 polyunsaturated fatty acids 1 gram daily *vs* placebo to standard therapy reduced the relative risk of all-cause mortality by 9% (p = 0.041) and the relative risk of death or admission to hospital for cardiovascular reasons by 8% (p = 0.009).

Ivabradine

■ Ivabradine does not modify the cardiac prognosis in patients with stable ischemic heart disease and left ventricular systolic dysfunction, but decreases the incidence of coronary events in the subgroup of subjects with a heart rate ≥ 70 bpm.

■ This has been recently shown by the **BEAUTIFUL** study (see p. 81).

Improved follow-up

Correction of anemia

■ Patients hospitalized for chronic heart failure often have a hemoglobin level of about 12 g/dL, corresponding to the lower limit of normal in adults.

■ This anemia has a multifactorial etiology: poor nutrition, hemodilution, associated renal failure inducing decreased erythropoietin levels, bone marrow depression, gastrointestinal bleeding related to aspirin therapy.

■ This anemia must be corrected.

■ Anemia has now been demonstrated to be an independent risk factor for death in patients with heart failure.

■ Retrospective analysis of the data of the **SOLVD** study (see p. 141) showed that a 1% reduction of hematocrit increased the relative risk of all-cause mortality.

■ In the population study conducted by **Ezekowitz** in Canada on 12,065 patients (median age: 78 years) hospitalized between 1993 and 2001 for recent heart failure, anemia was detected in 17% of cases and was accompanied by an increased risk of death.

■ Correction of even moderate anemia accompanying heart failure by erythropoietin (EPO) and iron significantly improves left ventricular function and NYHA class.

■ This was demonstrated for the first time by the study by **Silverberg** conducted in 32 patients with a mean age of 73.5 years with chronic heart failure (NYHA class III-IV; ventricular ejection fraction ≤ 40%) and a hemoglobin level permanently between 10.0 and 11.5 g/dL. SC injection of EPO (4,000 IU/week or if necessary 2 to 3 times per week) and IV administration of iron (200 mg in 150 ml of normal saline over 60 minutes every 2 weeks to increase hemoglobin to at least 12.5 g/dL) *vs* standard therapy improved NYHA class by 42.1% (*vs* 11.4% alteration), increased left ventricular ejection fraction by 5.5% (*vs* 5.4% reduction) and decreased the number of days of hospitalization by 79.0% (*vs* 57.6% increase), with a mean follow-up of 8.2 ± 2.6 months.

■ The effect of erythropoietin on the morbidity and mortality of patients with chronic heart failure and left ventricular ejection fraction ≤ 35% and anemia is currently under evaluation (**RED-HF** study).

Follow-up based on BNP levels

■ A treatment strategy systematically designed to achieve marked reduction of BNP levels ensures more marked reduction of morbidity and mortality than follow-up based on clinical findings alone.

■ This was demonstrated by the **STARS BNP** study conducted in 220 patients with chronic heart failure (NYHA class II-III) receiving optimal therapy, with a median follow-up of 15 months, more intense therapy, essentially higher doses of ACE inhibitors and beta-blockers designed to achieve BNP < 100 pg/ml, *vs* standard therapy significantly decreased the incidence of the primary endpoint (death or hospitalizations related to heart failure) observed in 24% *vs* 52% of cases (p < 0.001).

■ This may be not the case in patients over the age of 75.

■ In the **TIME-CHF** study conducted in 499 symptomatic patients hospitalized for an acute episode of heart failure during the previous year, stricter therapy based on monitoring of BNP levels *vs* standard therapy guided by symptoms, decreased mortality and hospitalizations for cardiac reason in patients aged 64 years to 75 years (mean age: 69 years) with a follow-up of 18 months but was not effective patients over the age of 75 (mean age: 82 years) in whom quality of life deteriorated.

Multidisciplinary global management

■ Global management of heart failure in an approach involving medical and paramedical personnel after the patient's return home improves quality of life and decreases the readmission rate.

■ This was demonstrated by the **AUCKLAND-HF, TEN-HMS** and **DIAL** randomized trials.

■ The effect of this integrated management on morbidity and mortality has not been formally demonstrated.

■ In the **COACH** study conducted in 1023 patients with a follow-up of 18 months, surveillance in the context of a community care/hospital network with the intervention of a nurse specifically devoted to this task *vs* conventional management did not appear to be more effective to reduce morbidity and mortality.

Cardiac resynchronization therapy

■ In about one-third of cases, chronic heart failure (NYHA class III-IV; left ventricular ejection fraction < 35%; left ventricular end-diastolic diameter ≥ 55 mm) is complicated by cardiac desynchronization, i.e. the various parts of the heart no longer contract synchronously during systole.

■ Desynchronization can be atriobiventricular, interventricular or intraventricular. Desynchronization is identified by widening of QRS complexes (> 0.12 s) on the surface ECG (The **RETHINQ** and **PROSPECT** studies showed that resynchronization is not beneficial in patients with QRS < 120 ms) and is confirmed by 2D echocardiography.

■ It is now demonstrated that desynchronization worsens symptoms, accelerates progression of left ventricular dysfunction and increases the risk of morbidity and mortality.

■ Cardiac desynchronization does not respond to any pharmacological treatment and can only be corrected by cardiac resynchronization by atriobiventricular pacing.

■ Cardiac resynchronization therapy is not designed to increase cellular contractility, but to control the sequences of left ventricular segmental contraction cycle by cycle in order to increase global contractility.

◆ *In practice, cardiac resynchronization therapy is indicated in patients with severe chronic heart failure not controlled by optimal medical therapy and presenting desynchronization of cardiac contraction documented by a QRS ≥ 120 ms.*

■ Cardiac resynchronization by multisite stimulation improves symptoms, quality of life and exercise capacity.

■ This was demonstrated by the European **MUSTIC** study and the American **MIRACLE** and **PATH-CHF II** studies, which demonstrated improvement of symptoms (reduction of NYHA class) and quality of life and exercise capacity scores. However, the very short follow-up (3 to 6 months) of these studies prevented any conclusions concerning the effect of cardiac resynchronization therapy on morbidity and mortality.

■ This beneficial effect is due to reduction of cardiac volume, especially left ventricular end-diastolic volume, attenuation of functional mitral incompetence and increased left ventricular ejection fraction, reflected by reduction of the levels of markers of heart failure (BNP, NT pro-BNP).

■ Cardiac resynchronization therapy by multisite stimulation reduces mortality.

■ This was authoritatively demonstrated by the **CARE-HF** study, thereby confirming the non-significant tendency revealed by the meta-analysis by **Bradley** and the **COMPANION** study.

■ In the **CARE-HF** study conducted in 813 patients with dilated cardiomyopathy (primary: 60%; ischemic: 40%) (left ventricular end-diastolic diameter indexed to height ≥ 30 mm/m) and systolic dysfunction (left ventricular ejection fraction $\leq 35\%$) with severe chronic heart failure (NYHA class III-IV), in sinus rhythm with QRS > 150 ms or > 120 ms but associated with at least 2 echocardiographic parameters of ventricular desynchronization, all receiving optimal medical therapy with a mean follow-up of 29.4 months, insertion of multisite stimulation associated with medical therapy compared to medical therapy alone significantly reduced the relative risk of the primary endpoint comprising total mortality and emergency hospitalization for major cardiovascular event by 37% ($p < 0.001$) and the relative risk of total mortality by 36% ($p < 0.002$), which constitutes a spectacular 10% reduction of the absolute risk of death.

■ The **REVERSE** study showed that cardiac resynchronization had a comparable beneficial effect in patients with severe heart failure (NYHA class III-IV) and in patients with asymptomatic or minimally symptomatic less severe heart failure (NYHA class I-II).

Implantable cardioverter-defibrillator (ICD)

■ Implantable cardioverter-defibrillator is recommended to improve the survival of patients who have survived cardiac arrest or with poorly tolerated sustained ventricular tachycardia or accompanied by left ventricular systolic dysfunction.

◆ *This was demonstrated by the* **MADIT** *and* **MUSTT** *studies conducted in patients with coronary heart disease with left ventricular dysfunction and severe spontaneous or electrically induced ventricular arrhythmias.*

■ In the **MADIT** study, ICD *vs* medical therapy significantly decreased the relative risk of total mortality by 54% (p = 0.009).

■ In the **MUSTT** study, ICD *vs* absence of ICD decreased the relative risk of cardiac arrest or arrhythmic mortality by 76% (p < 0.001).

■ Implantation of an ICD (at least 40 days after acute myocardial infarction) is a reasonable option to reduce the incidence of sudden death in selected patients with left ventricular ejection fraction < 30-35% who remain symptomatic despite optimal medical therapy.

■ This was demonstrated by the **MADIT II** study, in which ICD combined with conventional medical therapy *vs* medical therapy only decreased the risk of death by 31%, corresponding to an absolute risk reduction of 3%.

■ This was confirmed by the **SCD-HeFT** study conducted in 2,521 patients with heart failure (NYHA class II-III; left ventricular ejection fraction ≤ 35%) receiving optimal medical therapy, in whom ICD *vs* placebo and amiodarone reduced the risk of death by 23% (p = 0.007) with a mean follow-up of 45.5 months.

■ However, it must be stressed that this result was achieved at the price of numerous potential complications and a cost/efficacy ratio that was probably lower than that reported.

◆ *In practice, there is no way, at the present time, to formally identify those patients with heart failure most likely to obtain a real benefit from ICD as primary prevention.*

Surgical treatment

■ Surgery should be considered when symptomatic heart failure is associated with anatomical lesions accessible to surgical repair.

Myocardial revascularization

■ Percutaneous or surgical myocardial revascularization procedures cannot be routinely recommended in the treatment of heart failure.

■ No data derived from large-scale multicenter trials have demonstrated that myocardial revascularization can improve the symptoms of heart failure.

Mitral valve surgery

■ Surgical correction of severe mitral incompetence related to ventricular dilatation can improve symptoms in selected patients already presenting severe left ventricular dysfunction.

■ This was demonstrated by observational studies conducted in patients with end-stage heart failure with a follow-up of up to 5 years.

Ventricular reconstruction

This procedure is designed to reduce the degree of cardiomegaly, which increases wall tension and oxygen consumption.

Excision of a left ventricular aneurysm

■ Left ventricular aneurysmectomy is indicated when heart failure is secondary to aneurysm.

Cardiomyoplasty

■ Cardiomyoplasty can only be recommended for the treatment of heart failure.

■ This technique has only been performed in a limited number of patients and is still under evaluation.

Left ventricular reduction surgery (Batista procedure)

■ Left ventricular reduction surgery cannot be recommended for the treatment of heart failure.

■ Left ventricular reduction surgery alone or combined with mitral surgery was recommended in the treatment of end-stage heart failure several years ago and raised great hopes. However, in view of the high failure rate, heart transplantation is subsequently required in many of these cases.

Heart transplantation

Although no large-scale controlled clinical trials have been conducted on heart transplantation, it now constitutes one of the treatment options for end-stage heart failure.

■ In correctly selected patients, heart transplantation, compared to conventional medical therapy, significantly increases survival, exercise capacity, return to work and quality of life.

■ The 5-year survival on immunosuppressive therapy is now estimated to be 70-80% and, in the best series, 66% of patients return to work either full-time or part-time by the end of the first year.

■ Apart from the problem of the shortage of donors, the major problem of heart transplantation is that of rejection, responsible for a considerable number of deaths during the first postoperative year. In the longer term, the prognosis can also be threatened by the consequences of immunosuppressive therapy (infection, hypertension, renal failure, neoplasm) and by the development of coronary disease in the transplant.

Artificial heart and ventricular assistance

■ At the present time, biventricular assistance can only be performed by means of external pumps; it can only be temporary (several months) because of the risk of infection.

■ Implantable systems are used increasingly often, but infectious and thromboembolic complications still limit their widespread use.

■ These techniques are indicated while waiting for heart transplantation in patients with severe acute myocarditis and in some patients requiring permanent hemodynamic assistance.

■ The **REMATCH** study conducted in 129 patients with end-stage heart failure (NYHA class IV; mean left ventricular ejection fraction: $17 \pm 5\%$) and ineligible for heart transplantation, implantation of an artificial heart compared to optimal medical therapy decreased the relative risk of all-cause mortality by 48% ($p = 0.001$), but with a 2.35-fold increase of serious adverse events, mostly infections, bleeding and equipment failure, with a follow-up of 2 years.

Ultrafiltration

■ Dialysis can be used in some cases of severe congestive heart failure refractory to diuretics.

■ Unfortunately, the improvement observed is only transient in most cases and it has not been demonstrated to improve prognosis.

Strength of recommendations

- **Class 1**   Evidence and/or general agreement that a given diagnostic procedure or treatment is beneficial, useful and effective.
- **Class 2**   Conflicting evidence and/or a divergence of opinion about the usefulness/efficacy of the treatment.
  - **Class 2a**   Weight of evidence/opinion is in favor of usefulness/efficacy.
  - **Class 2b**   Usefulness/efficacy is less well established by evidence/opinion.
- **Class 3**   Evidence or general agreement that the treatment is not useful/effective and in some cases may be harmful.

Strength of evidence

- **Strength of evidence A**   Data derived from at least two randomized clinical trials or meta-analyses.
- **Strength of evidence B**   Data derived from a single randomized trial or from non-randomized studies.
- **Strength of evidence C**   Consensus opinion of the experts and/or small studies, retrospective studies or registries.

Stages of heart failure
(New York Heart Association [NYHA] classification)

- **Class I**   • No limitation of physical activity. Ordinary physical activity does not cause undue fatigue, palpitation, or dyspnea.
- **Class II**   • Slight limitation of physical activity. Comfortable at rest, but ordinary physical activity results in fatigue, palpitation, or dyspnea.
- **Class III**   • Marked limitation of physical activity. Comfortable at rest, but less than ordinary activity causes fatigue, palpitation, or dyspnea.
- **Class IV**   • Unable to carry out any physical activity without discomfort. Symptoms of cardiac insufficiency at rest. If any physical activity is undertaken, discomfort is increased.

Measurement of left ventricular ejection fraction (LVEF)

- Left ventricular ejection fraction is determined by:

$$\text{LVEF} = \frac{V_{ed} - V_{es}}{V_{ed}} \times 100 = \frac{SV}{V_{ed}} \times 100$$

Its normal value is $\geq 60\%$.

V_{ed}: end-diastolic volume; V_{es}: end-systolic volume;   SV: stroke volume.

Heart failure with preserved systolic function
(so-called diastolic heart failure)

1) Heart failure with preserved systolic function (left ventricular ejection fraction > 45-50%) represents 50% of all cases of heart failure and has the same annual survival rate as heart failure related to systolic dysfunction.

2) Pathophysiologically, it is essentially due to increased left ventricular end-diastolic pressure.

3) It is particularly frequent in the elderly and is often accompanied by HT, LVH, and hypertrophic cardiomyopathy.

4) The diagnosis of heart failure with preserved systolic function is based on the presence of 3 criteria (European Society of Cardiology, *Eur Heart J* 1998; 19:990-1003):
– symptoms or signs of heart failure;
– normal or only slightly altered left ventricular systolic function;
– presence of abnormalities of left ventricular relaxation, filling and diastolic compliance.

5) In his general review, **de Groote** (*Arch Cardiovasc Dis* 2008; 101:361-372) reported that only 3 clinical trials have specifically evaluated the impact of various drug classes on morbidity and mortality: **DIG** digoxin; **CHARM-preserved**, ARA 2 (candesartan), **PEP-CHF**, ACE inhibitor (perindopril). The results were disappointing, as none of the drug classes studied significantly improved the prognosis of the disease.

6) In practice, the treatment of heart failure with preserved systolic function is therefore schematically based on the same medications as those used for systolic heart failure, but with a few minor changes:
– diuretics and nitrates must be used cautiously to avoid any risk of hypovolemia and hypotension;

– positive inotropic agents, especially cardiac glycosides, should not be used, although they can sometimes be useful to slow the heart rate during an episode of acute heart failure.

CHAPTER 9

Atrial fibrillation

Antiarrhythmic therapy

Cardioversion for atrial fibrillation (AF)

■ In very recent AF (≤ 48 hours), sinus rhythm returns spontaneously in about one half of cases and IV digoxin does not have a significant effect on the reduction rate.

■ This was the conclusion of the **DAAF** study, which included 239 patients with AF lasting ≤ 7 days (mean duration: 22 hours). Digoxin *vs* placebo did not modify the reduction rate at the 16th hour (51% *vs* 46%), but significantly slowed the heart rate of AF by the 2nd hour.

■ Classically, pharmacological or electrical cardioversion must be preceded by effective anticoagulation for at least 3 weeks.

■ This prolonged anticoagulation is not essential when AF is very recent or when transesophageal echocardiography (TEE) confirms the absence of left atrial thrombosis.

■ This was demonstrated by the **ACUTE** study conducted in 1,222 patients with AF for more than 2 days (median duration: 13 days). The TEE-guided approach (brief anticoagulation before electrical cardioversion in the absence of atrial thrombus, continued for 4 weeks after cardioversion) compared to the conventional strategy (oral anticoagulant therapy for

3 weeks preceding electrical cardioversion and continued for 4 weeks after return of sinus rhythm) did not modify the embolic event rate at 8 weeks (0.81% *vs* 0.50%), while decreasing bleeding complications and increasing the sinus rhythm restoration rate after electrical cardioversion (71.1% *vs* 65.2%; p = 0.03).

■ Although external electrical cardioversion (EEC) is usually more effective, pharmacological cardioversion can be attempted in AF present for less than 7 days.

■ Several small studies have demonstrated the efficacy of a loading dose of amiodarone and class Ic antiarrhythmics, with a cardioversion rate as high as 80% when AF was present for less than 48 hours.

■ In the meta-analysis by **Chevalier** based on 13 studies comprising 1,174 patients with AF present for less than 7 days, the cardioversion rate at the 24th hour was similar with amiodarone and class Ic antiarrhythmics and significantly superior to that obtained with placebo.

■ Impregnation with antiarrhythmic drugs increases the chances of immediate success of electrical cardioversion and reduces the risk of early recurrence of AF.

Prevention of recurrent atrial fibrillation

■ Not all cases of reduced AF require long-term antiarrhythmic therapy.

■ This is the case of a first episode of well tolerated AF in a patient with a healthy heart in the presence of a cardiac or non-cardiac predisposing factor that can be eliminated or treated (acute alcoholism, electrocution, hyperthyroidism, acute pulmonary disease, acute pericarditis, acute myocardial infarction, acute myocarditis, cardiac surgery).

■ The efficacy of beta-blockers and heart-rate-lowering calcium channel blockers has not been clearly demonstrated.

■ Amiodarone is more effective than sotalol and class I antiarrhythmics.

 ■ This was demonstrated by the **CTAF** studies, a predefined analysis of the **AFFIRM** study and the **SAFE** study.

■ The choice of antiarrhythmic depends on the risk/benefit balance which must be evaluated according to age, presence or absence of heart disease and its severity, severity of the symptoms, and the presence of conduction disorders on ECG.

 ■ Amiodarone must not be systematically prescribed as first-line therapy.

 ■ Only amiodarone is recommended in patients with heart failure.

 ■ In patients with stable ischemic heart disease without heart failure, sotalol should be used as first-line therapy and amiodarone as second-line therapy, while avoiding class I antiarrhythmics.

 ■ Class Ia antiarrhythmics (quinidine) and sotalol should not be used in patients with HT and LVH because of the risk of torsades de pointes.

■ Endocavitary radiofrequency ablation is very promising.

 ■ The best indication is symptomatic and frequent paroxysmal AF refractory to at least two antiarrhythmic drugs. Improvement of the technique allows extension of the indications with success rates > 50%.

■ Totally asymptomatic recurrences of AF during antiarrhythmic therapy are very frequent.

 ■ This was demonstrated by the **PAFAC** study conducted in 848 patients, in which 70% of all recurrences of AF were completely asymptomatic (detection by daily telephone transmission of the ECG).

■ ACE inhibitors and ARBs are effective to prevent atrial fibrillation.

■ This was the conclusion of the meta-analysis by **Healey** based on 11 studies comprising 56,308 patients. Globally, ACE inhibitors and ARBs decreased the relative risk of AF by 28% (p = 0.0002) with a similar effect of the 2 drug classes and a more marked effect in studies conducted in patients with heart failure (44% reduction of the relative risk; p = 0.007).

Slowing of heart rate in atrial fibrillation

■ Pharmacological treatment is designed to slow heart rate to 60-80 bpm at rest and 90-115 bpm on moderate exercise.

■ Digoxin is rarely sufficient to slow heart rate on exercise and beta-blockers, diltiazem or verapamil are necessary in the case of persistent palpitations on exercise in the absence of congestive heart failure.

Control of sinus rhythm *vs* control of ventricular rate

■ In persistent AF at high risk of recurrence and/or stroke, the strategy of maintaining sinus rhythm at all costs does not provide any obvious benefit and could even be harmful.

■ This was the conclusion of 3 small morbidity and mortality studies (**PIAF**, **RACE** and **STAF**), and especially the **AFFIRM** mortality study.

■ The **AFFIRM** study included 4,060 patients with a mean age 70 years at high risk of stroke (ischemic heart disease and/or hypertension present in 88% of cases, left atrial dilatation present in 65% of cases and left ventricular systolic dysfunction present in 26% of cases), with recurrent AF in 2/3 of cases.

– After 5 years, 34.6% of patients in the heart rate control group and 62.6% of patients in the rhythm control group were in sinus rhythm, after one or several cardioversions if necessary and an antiarrhythmic (amiodarone in 2/3 of patients). Permanent anticoagulation (INR between 2 and 3) was also mandatory in the heart rate control group and strongly recommended in the rhythm control group, in which it was administered in about 70% of patients.

– At 5 years, total mortality tended to be higher in the rhythm control group (23.8% *vs* 21.3%; p = 0.08). The ischemic stroke rate was low and identical in the 2 groups (1% per year), and stroke mainly occurred in the case of absent or insufficient anti-coagulation. The rhythm control strategy induced more adverse drug effects and hospitalizations, without improving the patients' quality of life.

■ In the majority of cases, apparent maintenance of sinus rhythm does not justify discontinuation of anticoagulation.

■ In the **AFFIRM** study, the ischemic stroke rate was low and identical (1% per year) in the rhythm control group and in the heart rate control group, but stroke mainly occurred in the case of absent or insufficient anticoagulation.

■ Control of sinus rhythm does not appear to be superior to control of ventricular rate in patients with heart failure over the age of 65.

■ This was the conclusion of the recent **AF-CHF** study which ran-domized 1,376 patients. With a mean follow-up of 37 months, control of sinus rhythm *vs* control of ventricular rate did not modify cardiovascular mortality (26.7% *vs* 25.2%; p = 0.59) or total mortality, or the incidence of stroke and deterioration of heart failure.

Antithrombotic therapy

■ Paroxysmal AF is associated with the same stroke risk as permanent AF and therefore requires the same anti-thrombotic therapy.

■ This was the conclusion of the **SPAF** program.

■ Aspirin prevents only 1 in 5 strokes.

■ This was the conclusion of the **AFASAK 1, SPAF 1** and **EAFT** studies and the **Atrial Fibrillation Investigators** meta-analysis.

■ Compared to placebo, oral anticoagulants (INR: 2-3) prevent 2 out of 3 strokes.

■ This was demonstrated by the meta-analysis by **Hart** based on the **AFASAK 1, SPAF 1, SPAF 2, BAATAF, CAFA, SPINAF** and **EAFT** studies, comprising a total of 2,900 patients with a mean age of 69 years, with HT in 45% of cases and a history of stroke in 45% and 20% of cases, respectively.

■ For a mean follow-up of 1.6 year, anticoagulation decreased the risk of all strokes by 62% in relative values and by 3.1% per year in absolute values, as well as total mortality by 26% in relative values and 1.6% per year in absolute values.

■ Compared to aspirin, oral anticoagulants (INR: 2-3) decrease the risk of ischemic stroke by one half.

■ This was the conclusion of the meta-analysis by **Van Walraven** based on the **AFASAK 1** and **2, PATAF, EAFT, SPAF 1, 2** and **3** studies, comprising a total of 4,052 patients with a mean age of 71.7 years. With a mean follow-up of 1.9 year, anticoagulation *vs* aspirin significantly decreased the risk of all strokes by 45%, the risk of ischemic stroke by 52% and the risk of cardiovascular events by 29%, without modifying total mortality, but by increasing the annual major bleeding rate (2.2% *vs* 1.3%; p = 0.02).

■ The superiority of oral anticoagulants compared to aspirin is all the more marked in patients with a higher thromboembolic risk.

■ According to the meta-analysis by **Hart**, anticoagulation *vs* aspirin can prevent 48 strokes per 1,000 patients treated in secondary prevention (history of stroke), 24 in primary prevention in patients with a high risk, 14 when the risk is considered to be moderate and only 4 in patients at low risk.

■ The combination of weak anticoagulation (INR: 1.2-1.5) and aspirin is insufficient in AF at high risk of stroke.

■ This was the conclusion of the **SPAF 3** study, which included 1,044 patients and which was prematurely suspended because of the much higher annual rate of stroke or embolic events with the weak anticoagulation plus aspirin combination compared to moderate anticoagulation alone (7.9% *vs* 1.9%; p < 0.0001).

■ The clopidogrel-aspirin combination is not sufficient in AF associated with at least a moderate risk of stroke.

■ This was the conclusion of the **ACTIVE W** study which included 6,706 patients. This study was prematurely terminated because the clopidogrel-aspirin combination *vs* anticoagulation by oral anticoagulants (INR 2-3) significantly increased the annual risk of events including stroke, noncerebral systemic embolism, myocardial infarction or vascular death (5.60% *vs* 3.93%, p = 0.0003).

■ The bleeding risk related to anticoagulants, although globally moderate, increases with age and level of anti-coagulation.

■ An INR value between 2 and 3 appears to be the best compromise to prevent stroke and limit the bleeding risk.
■ International guidelines consider that slightly weaker anti-coagulation (INR: 1.6 to 2.5) is acceptable in patients over the age of 75.

■ According to **international guidelines** (**ACC, AHA, ESC**), the choice between aspirin and oral anticoagulants depends on the risk of stroke.

■ Risk factors for stroke are classified as:
– major: history of stroke, TIA or arterial embolism, mitral stenosis, mechanical valvular prosthesis;
– moderate: age ≥ 75 years, HT, diabetes, heart failure, LVEF ≤ 35%;
– minor: age between 65 and 74 years, female gender, ischemic heart disease, thyrotoxicosis.
■ Oral anticoagulants are recommended in the presence of a major factor or when a moderate factor is associated with any other risk factor.
■ Aspirin is recommended in the absence of a major or moderate risk factor.
■ Either aspirin or oral anticoagulants can be used in patients with not more than one moderate risk factor.

Classification of atrial fibrillation
(*Circulation* 2001; *104*: 2118-2150)

- **Recurrent AF**: Two or more episodes of AF

- **Paroxysmal AF**: Spontaneously resolving AF, generally lasting less ≤ 7 days and usually ≤ 24 h

- **Persistent AF**: Sustained AF (usually lasting > 7 days), in which reduction is obtained (or attempted) by electrical or pharmacological cardioversion

- **Permanent AF**: Long-standing AF for which cardioversion has failed or was not attempted

- **Nonvalvular AF**: No mitral stenosis or prosthetic heart valve

- **Lone AF**: No clinical or echocardiographic evidence of cardiopulmonary disease

Bleeding risk with oral anticoagulants – Beyth's score
(*Am J Med* 1998; *105*: 91-99)

• Age > 65 years	1 point
• History of gastrointestinal bleeding	1 point
• History of stroke	1 point

• One or more of the following diseases:
    - recent myocardial infarction
    - hematocrit < 30%
    - renal insufficiency
    - diabetes
	1 point

Risk level	4-year incidence of major bleeding
• **Low** (score = 0 point)	3%
• **Moderate** (score = 1-2 points)	12%
• **High** (score = 3-4 points)	53%

The main factors responsible for major bleeding are oral anticoagulant overdose and concomitant use of non-steroidal anti-inflammatory drugs.

CHAPTER 10

Venous thromboembolism

Deep vein thrombosis

Primary prevention

■ Unfractionated heparin (UFH) prescribed preventively by SC injection during the perioperative period decreases the incidence of venous thromboembolism.

■ This was demonstrated by the meta-analysis by **Collins** based on 74 trials comprising 15,598 patients, in which heparin decreased the frequency of asymptomatic deep vein thrombosis detected by labeled fibrinogen by 67% ± 4% and the risk of fatal or nonfatal pulmonary embolism by 64% ± 15%.

■ Low molecular weight heparins (LMWH) are as safe and as effective as unfractionated heparin in primary prevention of deep vein thrombosis.

■ This was demonstrated by the meta-analyses of **Nurmohamed** and **Leizorovicz**.

■ This was subsequently confirmed by the study by **Hull** conducted with logiparin, the study by **Kakkar** conducted with dalteparin, and the studies by **Bergqvist** and **Geerts** conducted with enoxaparin.

■ In the particular case of long-haul flights (lasting 10 to 15 hours), the use of compression stockings and/or enoxaparin injection (single SC injection of 1,000 IU [0.1 ml/

10 kg] 2 to 4 hours before the flight) significantly lowers the risk of deep vein thrombosis.

- This was demonstrated by the **LONFLIT II** and **III** studies.

■ Fondaparinux, a synthetic pentasaccharide and an indirect inhibitor of activated factor X (Xa), administered by subcutaneous injection, has been shown to be more effective and just as safe as enoxaparin for primary prevention of venous thromboembolism after orthopedic surgery.

- This was demonstrated by the **PENTHIFRAS** study conducted in 1,711 patients, the **PENTAMAKS** study conducted in 724 patients, the **EPHESUS** study conducted in 2,309 patients and the **PENTATHLON** study conducted in 227 patients.
- Unlike heparin, it does not act on platelets, eliminating the need to monitor platelet counts.

■ Rivaroxaban, an orally-active direct factor Xa inhibitor, is significantly more effective and just as safe as enoxaparin for prevention of venous thromboembolic events related to orthopedic surgery.

- This was demonstrated by the **RECORD 1, 2** and **3** studies conducted in 4,541, 2,509 and 2,531 patients operated for total hip replacement (**RECORD 1 and 2**) or total knee replacement (**RECORD 3**), respectively. Oral rivaroxaban 10 mg daily initiated 6 to 8 hours after closing the incision vs a single daily dose of enoxaparin 40 mg SC initiated 12 hours before surgery then resumed 6 to 8 hours after closing the incision, significantly reduced the incidence of the primary composite endpoint (symptomatic or asymptomatic deep vein thrombosis, subsequently demonstrated by bilateral venography, nonfatal pulmonary embolism, all-cause mortality) in each of the 3 studies: 1.1% vs 3, 7% ($p < 0.001$); 2.0% vs 9.3% ($p < 0.0001$); 9.6% vs 18% ($p < 0.001$), respectively, and decreased the incidence of the secondary composite endpoint comprising major thromboembolic events (deep vein thrombosis, nonfatal pulmonary embolism, thromboembolic death): 0.2% vs 2.0% ($p < 0.001$); 0.6% vs 5.1% ($p < 0, 0001$); 1.0% vs 2.6% ($p = 0.01$), respectively. The incidence of all bleeding (about 5 to 6%) and major bleeding (about 0.5%) was similar with rivaroxaban and enoxaparin.

■ In the **RECORD 4** study (total knee replacement), rivaroxaban 10 mg daily *vs* a higher dosage of enoxaparin (30 mg twice daily) nevertheless significantly reduced the thromboembolic risk by 31%.

◆ *Following withdrawal of ximelagatran from the market, due to the development of serious hepatic adverse effects, direct inhibitors of factor Xa (apixaban, dabigatran [in the RENOVATE study, it was shown to be noninferior to enoxaparin], razaxaban) are continuing to be developed. The MAGELLAN (prevention of thromboembolism in medically ill patients), EINSTEIN (treatment of acute thromboembolism), ROCKET AF (prevention of systemic arterial embolism in AF not related to valvular heart disease), and ATLAS ACS TIMI 46 (treatment of acute coronary syndromes) studies are underway with rivaroxaban.*

■ Aspirin, administered at a dosage of 75-150 mg daily to patients with a high cardiovascular risk, provides less effective prophylaxis of venous thromboembolism in medical or surgical settings.

■ In the **ATT** meta-analysis, platelet aggregation inhibitors decreased the risk of fatal or nonfatal pulmonary embolism by about 25% (0.46% *vs* 0.61%; $p < 0.01$).

■ In the **PEP** study conducted in 13,356 patients operated for hip fracture, aspirin 160 mg daily *vs* placebo initiated 5 weeks before the operation and continued, when possible, for 35 days postoperatively reduced the risk of pulmonary embolism by 43% ($p = 0.002$) and the risk of symptomatic deep vein thrombosis by 29% ($p = 0.03$).

Curative treatment

■ LMWH are at least as effective and safer than UFH in the curative treatment of venous thromboembolism.

■ This was demonstrated by several meta-analyses and numerous therapeutic trials conducted in patients with proximal or distal deep vein thrombosis, possibly associated with pulmonary embolism.

■ Except for particular cases (renal insufficiency, presence of bleeding or absence of clinical response), LMWH therapy does not require regular monitoring of clotting parameters.

■ Fondaparinux is not inferior to enoxaparin in terms of efficacy and is just as well tolerated.

■ This was shown in 2004 by the **MATISSE** study conducted in patients with symptomatic deep vein thrombosis.

■ Thrombolytic therapy is not routinely used in the presence of deep vein thrombosis.

■ Although it is more effective than conventional heparin therapy on the venous revascularization rate, it markedly increases the risk of major bleeding and pulmonary embolism.

■ This was demonstrated by the study by **Schweizer** conducted in 250 patients with a mean age of 40 years presenting acute deep vein thrombosis of the lower limb.

■ However, it may be justified in extreme limb-threatening thrombotic situations.

Secondary prevention

■ Anticoagulant treatment is remarkably effective in secondary prevention, but its optimal duration has not been clearly defined.

■ Prolonged prophylaxis (6 months) appears to be more effective than brief treatment (3 months) and the risk of recurrence after stopping oral anticoagulants is closely related to the presence or absence of a predisposing cause for the initial episode.

■ After proximal deep vein thrombosis, the use of compression stockings decreases the incidence of post-thrombotic syndrome by about 50% ($p < 0.001$).

■ This was demonstrated by the randomized trial by **Brandjes** conducted in 194 patients hospitalized for a first episode of proximal deep vein thrombosis of the lower limb, with a mean follow-up of 76 months.

Pulmonary embolism

Severity criteria

■ Classically, life-threatening pulmonary embolisms are anatomically massive (> 50% obstruction of pulmonary arteries or occlusion of at least 2 lobar arteries).

■ In fact, the hemodynamic instability secondary to right ventricular failure, dependent on the size of the embolus and the underlying cardiopulmonary state, is a much more reliable indicator of the severity of pulmonary embolism than the degree of angiographic obstruction.

■ For example, anatomically massive pulmonary embolism is not inevitably accompanied by shock and can have a good prognosis, while an anatomically less extensive pulmonary embolism can induce hemodynamic instability, or even death, if it occurs in a cardiorespiratory system altered by pre-existing disease.

■ The severity of pulmonary embolism is now defined by clinical signs.

◆ *According to the guidelines of the* **European Society of Cardiology** (Eur Heart J *2000*; 21: *1301-1336*):

■ Pulmonary embolism is described as massive when it is accompanied by shock or hypotension (systolic blood pressure ≤ 90 mmHg) or a pressure drop ≥ 40 mmHg for at least 15 minutes, if not caused by new-onset arrhythmia, hypovolemia or sepsis. It usually corresponds to vascular obstruction > 50%.

■ Pulmonary embolism is described as submassive when it is accompanied by normal blood pressure and clinical (jugular turgescence, hepatojugular reflux), hemodynamic (mean pulmonary artery pressure > 20 mmHg) or echocardiographic signs of right ventricular failure (right ventricular overload and/or pulmonary HT defined by a tricuspid jet velocity > 2.8 m/second). Ventricular dilatation is usually secondary to vascular obstruction ≥ 30%.

■ Pulmonary embolism is described as minor when it is accompanied by elevation of mean pulmonary artery pressure < 20 mmHg and does not induce any echocardiographic signs of right ventricular overload or dilatation. It usually corresponds to pulmonary vascular obstruction ≤ 20%.

Curative treatment

■ The studies by **Théry** and **Meyer** demonstrated that LMWH can replace UFH in the treatment of non-massive pulmonary embolism.

■ These preliminary studies were confirmed by the results of the **THÉSÉE** and **ACTS** studies conducted with tinzaparin and the **COLOMBUS** study conducted with reviparin.

■ Fondaparinux is as effective as UFH for initial treatment of hemodynamically stable pulmonary embolism.

■ This was demonstrated in 2003 by the **MATISSE** study conducted in 2,213 patients with symptomatic acute pulmonary embolism.

■ Intravenous thrombolysis or even immediate embolectomy are currently reserved for the treatment of massive pulmonary embolism defined clinically by poor hemodynamic tolerance, signs of right ventricular mechanical overload (dilatation of right chambers, elevation of BNP levels) or myocardial ischemia (elevation of troponin levels).

■ Massive pulmonary embolism corresponds to arterial obstruction > 50%. In these patients, the mortality is higher than 30% with heparin and IV thrombolysis (the 3 thrombolytics currently approved are streptokinase, urokinase and alteplase or tPA) is superior to heparin to ensure early pulmonary revascularization (40% to 50% relative gain in 12 to 24 hours) and a rapid reduction of pulmonary vascular resistance (30% to 40% reduction in less than 6 hours).

■ However, thrombolytic therapy is associated with an increased risk of major bleeding and only a large-scale randomized controlled trial would be able to definitively demonstrate its value in this indication.

Miller's index (*BMJ* 1971; 2: 681-687)

• Miller's index is used to evaluate the severity of pulmonary embolism by estimating the percentage of pulmonary vascular obstruction.
  It is calculated by attributing a peripheral pulmonary perfusion coefficient and a pulmonary artery obstruction coefficient.

The peripheral pulmonary perfusion coefficient is attributed to each of the six pulmonary territories according to the following score:
• normal blood supply = 0
• moderately decreased blood supply = 1
• severely decreased blood supply = 2
• total absence of blood supply = 3
  The left and right perfusion coefficient therefore varies between 0 and 9.

The pulmonary artery obstruction coefficient increases with the caliber of the artery blocked by the thrombus:
• pulmonary artery trunk = 16
• right pulmonary artery = 9
• left pulmonary artery = 7
• right upper lobe artery = 3
• culmen = 2
• middle lobe artery = 2
• lingula = 2
• right lower lobe artery = 4
• left lower lobe artery = 3
• segmental artery = 1 (9 arteries on the right and 7 on the left)
  The maximum obstruction coefficient is 9 on the right and 7 on the left.

The total score (perfusion coefficient + obstruction coefficient) therefore varies between 0 and 18 on the right and 0 and 16 on the left.

$$\text{Miller's index (\%)} = \frac{\text{perfusion coefficient} + \text{obstruction coefficient}}{34}$$

• Miller's index, commonly used in Europe, can overestimate the extent of pulmonary vascular obstruction in the case of massive embolism.

• Walsh's score (*Circulation* 1973;47 suppl. II:II-101) is more widely used in the United States, but does not take into account the alteration of peripheral perfusion.

Pulmonary embolism; essential concepts
European Society of Cardiology guidelines
(Eur Heart J 2000;21:1301-1336)

- Approximately 25% of patients with suspected pulmonary embolism will have the diagnosis refuted by a normal perfusion lung scan.

- A normal D-dimer level (< 500 ng/ml) measured by an ELISA assay may safely exclude pulmonary embolism.

- Ultrasonography shows a proximal deep vein thrombosis in 50% of patients with proven pulmonary embolism, but a normal examination does not rule out this diagnosis.

- Pulmonary embolism should be treated by IV infusion of unfractionated heparin at a dosage adjusted to the APTT; LMWH may be used in patients with non-massive pulmonary embolism.

- Oral anticoagulant treatment should be initiated during the first 3 days with an overlap with heparin therapy for 4 to 5 days. Heparin should be continued until the target INR (2.0-3.0) is obtained.

- Thrombolytics must only be used when the diagnosis of pulmonary embolism has been confirmed. They are indicated in massive pulmonary embolism, but their use in sub-massive pulmonary embolism is controversial.

- Dobutamine and dopamine may be used when pulmonary embolism is associated with low cardiac index and normal blood pressure and vasopressor drugs may be used in hypotensive patients.

Right heart thromboembolism
(Chest 2002;121:806-814)

- Right heart thromboembolism often corresponds to emboli in transit between peripheral deep veins and the pulmonary artery. They are situated in the right atrium or right ventricle; they are often mobile, forming serpiginous masses reflecting the morphology of the vein from which they are derived. The incidence of right heart thromboembolism could be close to 20% in patients with massive pulmonary embolism examined early in the course.

- In the retrospective analysis by **Rose** based on 95 publications published between 1996 and 2000 and comprising 177 cases of right heart thromboembolism associated with pulmonary embolism in 98% of cases:

  - the diagnosis of right heart thromboembolism was based on transthoracic (83.1% of cases) or transesophageal (14.1% of cases) echocardiography;

  - treatment comprised anticoagulants (19.8% of cases), thrombectomy (35.6%), and thrombolysis (35%);

  - the overall mortality rate was 27.1%. The mortality rate associated with anticoagulants, embolectomy, and thrombolysis was 28.6%, 23.8%, and 11.3%, respectively and 100% in the absence of treatment, reported in 9% of cases.

- Thrombolytic therapy was associated with a significantly improved survival rate (p < 0.05) compared to either anticoagulants or surgery. The major complication of thrombolytic therapy is significant bleeding, which occurs in as many as 20% of patients.

CHAPTER 11

Stroke

Primary prevention of atherothrombotic stroke or TIA

■ Stroke represents the third leading cause of mortality in the world after cardiovascular disease and cancer. Each year in the USA, more than 700,000 strokes are responsible for 150,000 deaths and 125,000 new cases of stroke are observed each year in France. The incidence of stroke increases exponentially with age: 1/1,000 before the age of 50 and 20/1,000 after the age of 80.

Control of cardiovascular risk factors

■ Control of HT and hypercholesterolemia ensures the best prevention of stroke.

■ For control of HT, see p. 15.

■ In terms of hypercholesterolemia, the meta-analysis by **Amarenco** based on 10 large-scale clinical trials (**ASCOT-LLA, ALLHAT-LLT, PROSPER, HPS, GREACE, MIRACL, LIPID, CARE, WOSCOPS, 4S)** and several small studies, comprising a total of almost 90,000 patients, showed that statins significantly lowered the risk of stroke by 21% (RR: 0.79 [0.73-0.85]), especially when LDL-C was decreased by 35 mg/L (about 1 mmol/L).

Antithrombotic therapy

Aspirin

■ In healthy subjects, aspirin has no effect on the risk of ischemic stroke, but significantly lowers the risk of nonfatal myocardial infarction, but with an increased bleeding risk.

- ■ This was demonstrated by the **BMD** and **PHS** studies.
- ■ This was confirmed by the meta-analyses by **Hennekens**, the **American Task Force** and **Eidelman.**
- – In the meta-analysis by **Eidelman** based on 5 trials comprising 55,580 subjects with a follow-up of 3.6 to 6 years, aspirin 75 to 500 mg daily *vs* placebo significantly decreased the relative risk of a first myocardial infarction by 32% and the relative risk of a vascular event by 15%, but had no significant effect on the risk of nonfatal stroke or vascular mortality.

■ In contrast, in high-risk subjects, aspirin significantly decreases the frequency of cardiovascular and cerebrovascular events, but is always associated with an increased bleeding risk.

- ■ In the **ATT** meta-analysis based on 287 studies comprising 212,000 high-risk patients as a result of their age or the presence of acute cardiovascular disease or predisposing factors, platelet aggregation inhibitor therapy, essentially aspirin 75-150 mg daily, *vs* placebo reduced the incidence of a serious vascular event comprising nonfatal myocardial infarction, nonfatal stroke or cardiovascular mortality by about 25%; aspirin also reduced the risk of each of these events by about 33%, 25% and 17%, respectively.

■ Prescription of aspirin as part of primary prevention must therefore be decided case by case.

- ■ According to the **European guidelines,** sufficient scientific data are not available to justify systematic prescription of aspirin to prevent stroke in asymptomatic subjects. However, aspirin can reduce the risk of myocardial infarction in this population. The final decision is therefore based on evaluation of each individual situation according to 3 facts that have now been clearly established, i.e. aspirin decreases the risk of coronary events, especially myocardial infarction, particularly in the presence of risk factors; it does not reduce the risk of ischemic stroke; it increases the bleeding risk and especially the risk of hemorrhagic stroke.

Primary prevention of embolic stroke

■ Many cardiac and aortic causes can be responsible for cerebral embolism (left atrial or ventricular thrombus, mitral valve disease, prosthetic heart valve, recent myocardial infarction, dilated cardiomyopathy, infectious endocarditis, patent foramen ovale, aneurysm of the interatrial septum, cardiac arrhythmias, aortic atheroma), but atrial fibrillation (AF), the most frequent cause, is the only cause to have been evaluated in large-scale clinical trials.

Oral anticoagulants

■ In patients with AF, anticoagulants significantly decrease the thromboembolic risk, especially the risk of cerebral thromboembolism.

■ This is particularly true when AF complicates the course of rheumatic heart disease, but it is also true when AF is not related to rheumatic heart disease.

■ Eight randomized trials have demonstrated the efficacy of warfarin *vs* placebo as primary prevention for thromboembolic stroke (**AFASAK 1, BAATAF, SPAF 1, CAFA, SPINAF, SPAF 2, SPAF 3** and **AFASAK 2**).

Aspirin

■ In the presence of AF unrelated to rheumatic heart disease, aspirin is less effective than anticoagulants in primary prevention of stroke.

■ In the **AFASAK 1** study, aspirin 75 mg daily behaved like placebo and did not significantly modify the number of thromboembolic events (essentially stroke) and vascular mortality.

■ In the **SPAF 1** study, aspirin 325 mg daily *vs* placebo decreased the rate of stroke, TIA and systemic embolism by only 44% (p < 0.01), while warfarin decreased this rate by 67% (p = 0.01).

■ The **SPAF 2** study reported similar results, as warfarin *vs* aspirin 325 mg daily reduced the risk of stroke by about 40%.

Secondary prevention of atherothrombotic stroke or TIA

■ In patients who have already had a stroke, the risk of death is higher in women (1 in 6) than in men (1 in 11) and about 1/3 of patients die within one year. In view of the severity of the physical and mental sequelae, 25 to 50% of survivors remain more or less dependent on another person for their daily activities. The 5-year risk of recurrence is about 30% and, in the longer term, the risk of mortality (especially cardiac mortality) is twofold higher than in the age-matched general population.

■ Secondary prevention of stroke is based on correction of cardiovascular risk factors, antithrombotic therapy and correction of a tight carotid artery stenosis in patients with TIA or minor stroke.

Control of risk factors

■ Blood pressure control after a stroke significantly reduces the recurrence rate.

■ This was suggested by data derived from the **INDANA** meta-analysis and the **PATS** study, in which not all patients were hypertensive.

■ This was confirmed by the **PROGRESS** double-blind study conducted in 6,105 hypertensive (48%) or non-hypertensive (52%) patients with a history, during the previous 5 years, of TIA or stroke without major disabling sequelae. With a follow-up of 4 years, active treatment including perindopril 4 mg daily possibly combined with indapamide 2-2.5 mg daily *vs* placebo in addition to conventional treatment significantly reduced the risk of another stroke (primary end-point) by 28% (p < 0.0001), the incidence of major cardiovascular events (vascular mortality, myocardial infarction and nonfatal stroke) by 26% (p < 0.001) and the incidence of dementia and cognitive disorders secondary to another stroke (secondary endpoints) by 34% and 45%, respectively.

■ In the **MOSES** study conducted in 1,405 hypertensive patients with a history of stroke or TIAs during the previous 2 years documented by brain CT or MRI, eprosartan 600 mg daily *vs* nitrendipine 10 mg daily, with a mean follow-up of 2.5 years, induced a similar reduction of BP to below 140/90 mmHg (in 75% of cases in the two groups) but more markedly reduced (by 21% [p = 0.014]) the incidence of the main composite endpoint comprising cardiovascular and cerebrovascular events and death; this result was due to a non-significant (p = 0.06) 25% reduction of cardiovascular events and a significant (p = 0.03) 25% reduction of cerebrovascular events.

■ In contrast, in the **PRoFESS** study which was conducted in 20,332 patients aged 55 years or older who had had an ischaemic stroke in the previous 90 days (in addition patients aged between 50 and 54 years or patients who presented 90 to 120 days after the qualifying stroke and who had two of the following additional risk factors: hyperlipidaemia, diabetes mellitus, hypertension, smoking, obesity [BMI ≥ 30], previous vascular disease [stroke, MI, or peripheral arterial disease], end-organ damage [retinopathy, left-ventricular hypertrophy, or microalbuminuria] were also recruted to the study), with a mean follow-up of 2.4 years, telmisartan 80 mg given once daily failed to prevent recurrent strokes (which occurred in 9% of patients in both the telmisartan and placebo groups) despite a 4 mmHg reduction of BP in comparison with placebo.

■ Aggressive reduction of cholesterol by atorvastatin significantly decreases the risk of recurrent stroke.

■ Up until now, the only available data were derived from the **HPS** study conducted in 20,536 patients at high cardiovascular risk, 3,200 of whom had had a stroke. In this group, with a follow-up of 5.5 years, simvastatin 40 mg daily *vs* placebo decreased the risk of a major coronary event, justifying the current AFSSAPS recommendations to prescribe a statin to all patients with a history of stroke. However, the statin had no effect on recurrent stroke, which was observed in 10.4% of cases (vs 10.5% with placebo), possibly because of the late inclusion of patients (an average of 4 to 6 years after the first stroke).

■ More recently, the **SPARCL** study conducted in 4,731 patients with stroke or TIA during the previous 6 months but free of coronary heart disease showed, for the first time, with a follow-up of 6 years, that addition of atorvastatin 80 mg daily vs placebo to optimal therapy including a platelet aggregation inhibitor (95% of cases) and an antihypertensive (68%), decreased the risk of another fatal or nonfatal stroke by 16% (p = 0.003) at the price of a slight but significant elevation of the risk of haemorrhagic stroke (RR: 1.66; p = 0.02). Remarkably, atorvastatin also decreased the risk of a major coronary event by 35% (p = 0.003) and the risk of all cardiovascular events by 26% (p < 0.001).

Platelet aggregation inhibitor monotherapy

■ After a first stroke or TIA, treatment with aspirin, dipyridamole or thienopyridines (ticlopidine, clopidogrel) significantly reduces the risk of recurrence.

◆ *Aspirin also reduces the incidence of myocardial infarction and vascular mortality and this beneficial effect outweighs the bleeding risk.*

■ This was demonstrated by the **CCS** study and the **SALT** study conducted in 585 patients and 1,360 patients with a history of cerebral or ocular TIA, respectively.

■ In the **ATT** meta-analysis based on 195 studies comprising 136,640 patients at high risk of vascular occlusion, platelet aggregation inhibitor therapy (essentially aspirin at the dosage of 75-325 mg daily) reduced the relative risk of non-fatal stroke by 25% (p < 0.0001), the relative risk of nonfatal or fatal ischemic stroke by 30% (p < 0.0001) and increased the relative risk of nonfatal or fatal cerebral hemorrhage by 22% (p < 0.01).

The beneficial effect of aspirin was largely counterbalanced by the increased risk of major extracranial bleeding, estimated to be about 1 to 2 additional cases per year per 1,000 patients treated.

■ In practice, aspirin is recommended at low dosages (50-325 mg daily), which are as effective as higher dosages but with better gastrointestinal safety.

■ This was demonstrated by the **UK-TIA, Dutch-TIA** and **ESPS 2** studies.

■ Dipyridamole prescribed alone or in combination with aspirin *vs* placebo was found to be effective for secondary prevention of atherothrombotic ischemic stroke in the **ESPS 2** study.

■ In the **ESPS 2** study conducted in 6,602 patients with a mean age of 67 years with a history of TIA or confirmed ischemic stroke during the previous 3 months, dipyridamole 400 mg daily *vs* placebo decreased the risk of stroke by 16.3% (p = 0.039), the combined risk of stroke or death by 15.4% (p = 0.015) and the risk of TIA by 18.3% (p < 0.01), with a follow-up of 2 years.

■ In this same study, the [aspirin 25 mg-dipyridamole 200 mg] combination twice daily *vs* placebo decreased the relative risk of stroke by 37.0% (p < 0.001), the combined risk of stroke or death by 24.4% (p < 0.001) and the risk of TIA by 35.9% (p < 0.001).

■ Ticlopidine and clopidogrel have been shown to be effective in secondary prevention of stroke.

■ In the **TASS** study and in the **CATS** study conducted in several thousand patients with a history of atherothrombotic stroke, ticlopidine 500 mg daily *vs* placebo (CATS study) or *vs* aspirin (TASS study) decreased the risk of nonfatal or fatal stroke by 21% to 23% (p = 0.02).

■ In the **CAPRIE** study conducted in 19,185 patients with a history of stroke, myocardial infarction or arterial disease of the lower limbs, clopidogrel 75 mg daily *vs* aspirin 325 mg daily globally decreased the relative risk of the composite endpoint comprising stroke, myocardial infarction or vascular mortality by 8.7% (p = 0.043), with a follow-up of 1.9 year.

Platelet aggregation inhibitor combination therapy

■ The aspirin-dipyridamole combination is more effective than aspirin alone.

■ In the **ESPS 2** study (see p. 189), the aspirin 25 mg-dipyridamole 200 mg twice daily combination *vs* aspirin 25 mg twice daily alone decreased the risk of recurrent neurological accidents by 18.1% (p = 0.013).

■ In the **ESPRIT** study conducted in 2,739 patients with a mean age of 63 ± 11 years with a history of stroke or TIA during the previous 6 months with no sequelae impairing their autonomy, with a mean follow-up of 3.5 years, the combination of aspirin 30 to 325 mg-dipyridamole 400 mg daily *vs* aspirin 30 to 325 mg daily alone, reduced the relative risk of the major events of the primary composite endpoint comprising vascular mortality, myocardial infarction or nonfatal stroke, and severe bleeding by 20% (RR: 0.80; [0.60-0.98]); surprisingly, severe bleeds were less frequent with combination therapy (35 *vs* 53).

■ These results were confirmed by the meta-analyses by **Leonardi-Bee** and **Thijs**.

■ The aspirin-dipyridamole combination is as effective as clopidogrel and this beneficial effect is not modified by the addition of telmisartan.

■ In the **PRoFESS** study conducted in 20,332 patients with a mean age of 66 years with an ischemic stroke during the previous 90 days, with a mean follow-up of 2.4 years, clopidogrel 75 mg daily and the combination of aspirin 25 mg-dipyridamole 200 mg twice daily exerted an equivalent effect on recurrent stroke, observed in 9% of cases in each treatment arm. No significant difference was observed between the 2 arms in terms of permanent disability and cognitive decline which were not modified by prophylaxis with telmisartan 80 mg daily (*vs* placebo).

■ The aspirin-clopidogrel combination is not more effective than aspirin or clopidogrel prescribed alone, but significantly increases the bleeding risk.

■ In the **MATCH** study conducted in 7,599 patients with recent stroke or TIA, with a follow-up of 18 months, the combination of aspirin 75 mg - clopidogrel 75 mg daily *vs* clopidogrel 75 mg daily did not modify the incidence of the primary composite endpoint comprising ischemic stroke, myocardial infarction, vascular mortality or readmission for acute ischemia (15.7% *vs* 16.7%; p = 0.24) but tripled the risk of major bleeding (1.9% *vs* 0.6%; p < 0.0001) and doubled the risk of life-threatening bleeding (2.6% *vs* 1.3%; p < 0.0001).

■ In the **CHARISMA** study conducted in 15,063 patients with a mean age of 64 years and presenting symptomatic (80% of cases) or asymptomatic (20%) cardiovascular disease or combining several risk factors, with a median follow-up of 28 months, the combination of aspirin 75-162 mg - clopidogrel 75 mg daily *vs* aspirin 75-162 mg daily did not significantly decrease the incidence of the primary composite endpoint comprising cardiovascular mortality, myocardial infarction and stroke (6.8% *vs* 7.3%; p = 0.22) but increased the rate of severe (1.7% *vs* 1.3%; p = 0.09) and moderate (2.1% *vs* 1.3%; p < 0.001) bleeding complications.

◆ *In summary, aspirin has been shown to be effective in the secondary prevention of stroke. Ticlopidine and clopidogrel are barely more effective than aspirin when all elements of the vascular prognosis are taken into account. The protective effect of dipyridamole appears to be additive to that of aspirin, but the superiority of this combination compared to aspirin alone was only demonstrated by the* **ESPS 2** *study. In practice, aspirin must be used alone as first-line therapy. In the case of recurrent stroke, aspirin is usually replaced by clopidogrel or dipyridamole is added. Clopidogrel is also used in patients not tolerating aspirin.*

Oral anticoagulants

■ Oral anticoagulants have not been shown to be more effective than aspirin in secondary prevention of atherothrombotic stroke (unrelated to cardiac embolism).

■ In the **WARSS** study conducted in 2,206 patients with ischemic stroke not related to cardiac embolism during the previous 3 days, with a mean follow-up of 10.2 ± 7.5 months, no significant difference was observed between warfarin (INR: 1.4-2.8) *vs* aspirin 325 mg daily in terms of the primary endpoint comprising ischemic stroke or all-cause mortality during the 2 years following randomization or in terms of the major bleeding risk which remained low.

Secondary prevention of embolic stroke

Oral anticoagulants

■ In patients with embolic stroke, especially in the presence of atrial fibrillation, oral anticoagulants significantly decrease the recurrence rate.

■ In the **EAFT** study conducted in 1,007 patients with atrial fibrillation unrelated to rheumatic heart disease and presenting a history of TIA or minor stroke during the previous 3 months, oral anticoagulants *vs* placebo significantly decreased the annual rate of major events, i.e. vascular mortality, nonfatal stroke, nonfatal myocardial infarction or systemic embolism by 47% (p = 0.001) and the annual rate of fatal or nonfatal stroke by 66% (p < 0.001). Oral anticoagulants have also been shown to be significantly more effective than aspirin in the prevention of major events, which were decreased by 40% (p = 0.008) especially due to a 62% reduction of nonfatal or fatal stroke (p < 0.001).

Correction of symptomatic carotid artery stenosis

■ When it is decided to perform a revascularization procedure, surgery remains the standard technique, as the noninferiority of angioplasty and stenting (*vs* surgery), in terms of mortality and stroke was not demonstrated by European **SPACE** and **EVA-3S** studies. Carotid angioplasty is therefore usually not indicated as first-line treatment.

■ Endarterectomy is very effective when carotid artery stenosis is symptomatic and very tight (≥ 85% according to the European evaluation [**ECST** study] and ≥ 70% according to the American evaluation [**NASCET** study]), as it significantly decreases the risk of ipsilateral stroke.

■ Endarterectomy is still effective, but to a lesser degree, when the symptomatic carotid artery stenosis is moderately tight (70-85% according to the European evaluation and 40-70% according to the American evaluation).

■ Endarterectomy is not indicated in patients with symptomatic but limited carotid artery stenosis, as the expected benefit does not counterbalance the operative risk.

   ◆ *According to* **Rothwell***, the benefit of surgery is greater in subjects over the age of 75 (vs younger than 65), especially males and when the procedure is performed less than 2 weeks after a TIA. According to* **Bond***, the estimated operative risk (death or stroke) of symptomatic carotid stenosis is 5.1%.*

   ■ These were the 3 conclusions reached by the **NASCET** and **ECST** studies.

■ Carotid angioplasty and stenting can be proposed in some cases.

   ■ For example in the case of surgical contraindications related to the patient's clinical (especially cardiorespiratory) or anatomical condition (tracheotomy, inaccessible stenoses, radiation stenoses, restenoses after surgery).

■ All these concepts are constantly evolving, especially due to technological progress.

   ■ In a recent meta-analysis of 5 trials comprising 2,122 patients, **Gurm** did not find any difference at 30 days between endarterectomy and carotid angioplasty and stenting in terms of mortality or stroke.

■ In the **SAPPHIRE** study conducted in 334 patients at high surgical risk and presenting a tight carotid stenosis, carotid angioplasty and stenting with the use of an emboli-protection device achieved comparable results at 3 years to those of endarterectomy in terms of the incidence of the primary composite endpoint comprising death, stroke and myocardial infarction.

■ Further information will be provided by the ongoing **CREST** and **ICSS** studies.

Correction of asymptomatic carotid artery stenosis

■ When asymptomatic carotid artery stenosis is ≥ 60% according to the European evaluation (≥ 25-30% according to American evaluation), the estimated annual risk of ipsilateral stroke is 2%.

■ The benefit of carotid endarterectomy is relatively low in this setting.

■ In the **ACST** study, endarterectomy compared to medical treatment reduced the annual stroke risk by only 1%.

■ This low benefit can only be achieved when a low operative risk (death and stroke) < 3% can be guaranteed.

■ The indication for endarterectomy must therefore be defined cautiously and must take into account the patient's age, the degree of stenosis and the surgeon's experience.

■ At the present time, there is no indication for angioplasty and stenting in asymptomatic carotid artery stenosis.

Index

Index of acronyms

Index of studies and meta-analyses

Imprimé dans l'UE

Mise en pages :
Compo-Méca s.a.r.l. – 64990 Mouguerre